HOW TO EAT

ANCIENT WISDOM FOR MODERN READERS

■ ■ ■

HOW TO EAT

■ ■ ■

An Ancient Guide for Healthy Living

A Buffet of Ancient Authors

Selected, translated, and introduced
by Claire Bubb

PRINCETON UNIVERSITY PRESS

PRINCETON AND OXFORD

Requests for permission to reproduce material from this work should be sent to permissions@press.princeton.edu

Published by Princeton University Press
41 William Street, Princeton, New Jersey 08540
99 Banbury Road, Oxford OX2 6JX

press.princeton.edu

All Rights Reserved

Library of Congress Cataloging-in-Publication Data

Names: Bubb, Claire, translator.
Title: How to eat : an ancient guide for healthy living : a buffet of
ancient authors / selected, translated, and introduced by Claire Bubb.
Description: Princeton ; Oxford : Princeton University Press, [2025] |
Series: Ancient wisdom for modern readers | Includes
bibliographical references. | Selection of works in Greek and
Latin with translation in English.
Identifiers: LCCN 2024023697 (print) | LCCN 2024023698 (ebook) | ISBN
9780691256993 (hardback) | ISBN 9780691261584 (ebook)
Subjects: LCSH: Diet—Mediterranean Region—Early works to 1800. |
Nutrition—Greece—Early works to 1800. | Nutrition—Rome—
Early works to 1800. | Food habits—Greece—Early works to 1800. | Food
habits—Rome—Early works to 1800. | Functional foods—
Early works to 1800. | BISAC: PHILOSOPHY / Social |
HEALTH & FITNESS / Diet & Nutrition / General
Classification: LCC TX360.M37 H67 2025 (print) |
LCC TX360.M37 (ebook) | DDC 613.209182/2—dc23/eng/20240819
LC record available at https://lccn.loc.gov/2024023697
LC ebook record available at https://lccn.loc.gov/2024023698

British Library Cataloging-in-Publication Data is available

Editorial: Rob Tempio and Chloe Coy

Production Editorial: Natalie Baan

Text Design: Pamela L. Schnitter

Jacket Design: Heather Hansen

Production: Erin Suydam

Publicity: Tyler Hubbert and Carmen Jimenez

Copyeditor: Hank Southgate

Jacket Credit: Still life, mosaic, 2nd century CE. From a villa at Tor Marancia,
near the Catacombs of Domitilla. Courtesy of Musei Vaticani.

This book has been composed in Stempel Garamond LT Std

Printed in the United States of America

1 3 5 7 9 10 8 6 4 2

CONTENTS

CONTENTS

CONTENTS

ILLUSTRATIONS

LIST OF ILLUSTRATIONS

ACKNOWLEDGMENTS

My thanks go first and foremost to Rob Tempio for tempting me to do this volume in the first place. It has been a delight. Thanks also to Ryan Bubb, Rhys Coiro, and Paul Starr for being early test readers and to Alexander Jones for orienting me properly to the Pleiades. I am also indebted to the anonymous referees for their helpful feedback and suggestions and to Chloe Coy, Natalie Baan, Hank Southgate, and everyone at Princeton University Press who worked to make this book a reality.

INTRODUCTION

Healthy eating is a perennially urgent topic. The modern eater is bombarded with dietary recommendations in various guises from almost every direction: doctors, cookbooks, weight-loss programs, government messaging, the media, food packaging, and all the corners of the Internet have urgent advice on what to eat, what *not* to eat, when, and how. Modern nutritional science is a comparatively new development. The modern vocabularies for the health consequences of food only began to emerge in the nineteenth and twentieth centuries: the idea of defining diet in terms of proteins, fats, and carbohydrates first entered the scene in the 1820s and '30s, and the term "vitamin" did not debut until 1912. Indeed, Michael Pollan's *In Defense of Food: An Eater's Manifesto* (Penguin, 2008) has popularly

problematized the lens of "nutritionism" through which the healthiness of today's food is gauged, framing it as a uniquely modern phenomenon. Yet, the reader of this book will find that this is not completely so. Many of the questions that so occupy the minds of today were equally salient to the ancient peoples of Greece and Rome, and many of their answers, though differing in their details, are resonant with our own.

Certainly, the specific terms and concepts by which today's doctors evaluate the healthiness and dietary suitability of our foods (vitamins, minerals, lipids, carbohydrates, protein, cholesterol, trans fats, calories, etc.)—not to mention the plethora of named and rule-bound ways of eating, whether medical or paramedical (the gluten-free diet, the low-FODMAP diet, the ketogenic diet, the paleolithic diet, and on nearly ad infinitum)—are all modern developments. Nevertheless, ancient Greco-Roman doctors were highly attuned to the variabilities among

foods and to the varying impacts that different diets exert on people's health. They discussed these variabilities at length, in theoretically sophisticated ways, with their own set of vocabulary for the differentiating qualities to be found in foods. And they developed detailed dietary recommendations, some examples of which are to be found in the following pages. Just like in the modern world, however, doctors did not have the monopoly on opinions about what makes a healthy diet. As everywhere, Greco-Roman food choices were equally imbued with moral and social dimensions. Though there was some fringe interest in vegetarianism, the moral dimension of food had much less to do with the foods themselves, and much more to do with the state of mind of the consumer: decadence and extravagance in the diet, as well as undue focus on the pleasures of food, were considered to betoken an unphilosophical lack of self-control. Likewise, there were social and cultural implications to many foods, sometimes

based on their price and attainability (Roman satirists found the contemporary craze for rare and fancy fish to have reached ridiculous proportions), sometimes related to their religious uses (a significant fraction of meat-eating was tied to religious animal sacrifice), sometimes on other grounds (the radish had associations with both rustic uncouthness and sexual debauchery). Nevertheless, the most voluble source of advice on how to eat in antiquity is the extensive medical literature on the subject, and it is texts from this body of writing that form the core of this volume.

Dietetics: Ancient Nutritional Science

From its very earliest written manifestations, Greek medicine focused on diet as a major pillar of health. Indeed, the author of the fifth-century BCE text *Ancient Medicine*, part of the canonical Hippocratic Corpus, equates the art of medicine with the art of nutrition: for him, medicine began when humans first learned how

to manipulate the nutritive capacity of foodstuffs through cooking and other forms of food preparation. Though Greek medicine also took recourse to surgical and pharmaceutical remedies, diet was the first line of attack, as well as the first line of defense. The reasons for this were both practical and theoretical. At a practical level, dietary changes were exponentially less risky than trying one's luck with medicinal plants or premodern surgical procedures—doctors and patients alike recognized this to be true. But diet also played a theoretically crucial role in ancient Greco-Roman understandings of health and the body, making its manipulation a scientifically credible therapeutic avenue.

Ancient medicine is a famously polyvocal space, so it is impossible to generalize completely, but there was a widespread understanding that whatever parts of ingested food were not excreted through the digestive system became assimilated to the body of the person who ate them—that is, that you quite literally

are what you eat. Similarly widespread was the idea that the human body is an amalgamation of different factors that are inherently in tension with one another and that must be kept in balance if the body is to remain healthy. Ultimately, these factors usually boil down to the elemental qualities of hot, cold, wet, and dry, but they also appear in the more corporeal guises of the humors—these were subsequently canonized as the familiar four (blood, phlegm, yellow bile, and black bile), but they were a more diverse and unruly bunch in the early centuries of Greek medical thought. The combined result of these two beliefs was the conviction that the qualities and attributes of the foods one consumes directly impact the quality and health of one's body. Not, in the end, a far cry from our modern beliefs, writ large.

Indeed, though the details are completely different and the research methodologies do not align, ancient discussion of the qualities of foods does not feel as foreign as it might, a fact stem-

ming largely from two common factors. First, setting aside their unfamiliar terms and categories, Greco-Roman thinkers shared our belief that there are things *in* our foods that affect our health. Granted, where we might say that something is full of vitamin C or a great source of protein, they instead describe foods as full of a drying power or a great source of nourishment. But the basic insight is the same: foods have largely invisible qualities within them that affect our bodies and that need to be explained to us by experts who have plumbed the depths of their natures. Second, and conversely, most of the foods that they are describing are foods that we still have an intimate and personal relationship to: we eat them. As a result, we directly experience how they make us feel. Here, the ancient sources are more explicit than we are used to our medical authorities being, but the things they describe are instantly recognizable. The ancient sources teem with descriptions of the experience of food: some foods go through

the bowels easily and rapidly, others tend toward constipation; some make you flatulent, others make you burp; some sit heavily on the stomach, others are refreshing. Indeed, as the late first-century CE Roman essayist Plutarch reminds us, you are the one with a front-row seat to your own digestion. He points out that paying as much attention to what a food makes you feel like as to what it tastes like will take you a long way toward finding your optimal diet, even without any medical advice: "it would be just as ridiculous to ask a doctor which foods are difficult or easy for you personally to digest, or which go through your bowels with difficulty and which easily, as it would be for you to inquire which are sweet and which are bitter or sour."[1]

This emphasis on careful observation of how food interacts with your body in real time feeds into the other major aspect of ancient dietetic advice: food choices are just one piece of the puzzle, which must be appropriately combined

with all the other aspects of a healthy lifestyle. The most obvious of these is exercise. Greco-Roman medical texts dilate at length on how to balance diet and exercise, both in terms of the quantities of each, but also in terms of their relative timing. In ancient dietetics, it makes a huge difference to the outcome for the body whether food precedes exertion or vice versa; advice in this regard will accordingly be different depending on whether you are trying to bulk up or lose a few pounds. Similarly, bathing was a major variable in ancient regimen, with its obvious potential for impact on one's balance of hot, cold, wet, and dry. Likewise, sleep habits, sex life, personal grooming, and even clothing selection all fell under the purview of dietetic advice. All of these daily lifestyle choices had implications for each other, and it was considered important to carefully calibrate these different activities with one's current bodily state and circumstances. Indeed, while many texts offer generalized advice, that advice

is always meant to be applied in a personalized and seasonally specific way: no two people should follow the exact same diet, nor should anyone stick unwaveringly to a single way of eating year-round. In fact, the seasonality of food choices is perhaps the hallmark of ancient dietetics. Dietary choices were seen as a powerful tool to counteract the changing effects on the body as the weather shifts from season to season and thus to maintain a healthy balance: in the cold and wet of winter, heating and drying foods keep your body from succumbing to phlegm, but they would be disastrously counterproductive in the hot, dry days of summer. But even within these guidelines, personalization is key, and a naturally dry person needs to calibrate differently than a naturally moist one does (likewise a young person versus an older one, a man versus a woman, etc.). Those with the money and the time were further encouraged to take this personalization down to the day or even the hour. It is a wise person who

keeps on eye on the state of their stomach and bowels and plans their day accordingly: better to stay in bed with a little indigestion than to proceed as usual and see it blossom into a more serious illness!

Indeed, all the dietetic advice discussed so far has been preventative. But when prophylactics failed and disease set in, diet was equally on the frontlines of medical treatment. In addition to these regimens for health, there were countless regimens for illness, each needing to be calibrated to the specific combination of disease and patient. In these situations, food was not merely nourishment, but effectively a medication. Indeed, there was no firm division between the categories of food and drug. Ancient doctors like Galen—whose works I have extensively drawn on in Part II—considered most foods to have certain potencies that could be harnessed to medical effect in the right situations. In fact, as we will see, lettuce—an unprepossessing vegetable to the modern eye—is his

prime example of something that is as much a drug as a food. This brings us back full circle to those invisible factors contained within foods: the juices, humors, and powers whose effects on the body the medical authors describe. Part II of this text offers examples of this advice about specific foods, so it seems advisable to turn now to providing some background for the broader food landscape within which these doctors were operating.

The Ancient Food Landscape

The "Mediterranean Diet" has become one of the most popular patterns for modern healthy eating since it was codified into a set of dietary guidelines in the mid-1990s. The ancient version and its modern namesake should not be assumed to perfectly align, but the "big three" will certainly be familiar: whole grains, olive oil, and wine. Wine is a huge topic of its own, which will appear only tangentially in the pages that follow—to do it justice would require a dedi-

cated book. Olive oil, too, while a major source of fat in ancient Greco-Roman diets, has a largely background role, as the vehicle, dressing, or cooking medium for the other foods in the spotlight (not to mention its frequent cameos as a moisturizer and bath soap). Grains, however, and their less glamorous companions the pulses (beans, lentils, etc.), will indeed be front and center: whether in the form of bread, savory cakes, porridge, or stews, they were the cornerstone of most simple meals. Vegetables and herbs, as well as meat and fish (usually in modest amounts, often preserved), enlivened these dishes and made for variety. Obviously, any generalization of this scale will obscure a huge range of regional idiosyncrasies. Culinary customs varied considerably over the geographical, chronological, and socioeconomic spans of the Greco-Roman world: where the classical Athenians had a soft spot for barley cakes, the imperial Romans had more of a love affair with wheaten bread; meanwhile in the Roman

provinces, the Gauls substituted butter for olive oil, while the Egyptians notoriously preferred beer to wine. Interestingly, though, there was a widespread view that lunch was optional—it was unremarkable to take only a single big meal, in the evening. This meal was usually some variation on the simple grain- or legume-based affair described above, but as the budget increased, so too did the complexity of the menu: we have copious evidence for extravagant, multicourse dinners with elaborately prepared and sometimes quite exotic dishes (which understandably exert a disproportionate pull on the modern imagination).[2]

When it comes to the ingredients for these meals, the food economy of the ancient Mediterranean was, unsurprisingly, less industrialized and more localized than today's. This manifested in a variety of ways. First, ancient eaters were much more attuned to the seasonality of food than the modern consumer. The lack of reliable refrigeration techniques limited the availability of fresh fruits and perishable vegetables to the

periods in which each one is ripe to be picked—sometimes a matter of a few weeks a year. As the entry on cucumbers in Part II suggests, only someone with the limitless resources and high-tech gadgetry of an emperor could hope to eat fresh produce out of its natural growing season. Animal-based foods were equally impacted: the availability of meats like beef and lamb, as well as the quality and abundance of fresh dairy products, were dependent on the annual breeding cycle of herd animals, a thought perhaps startling to the modern supermarket shopper. Even grains, with their longer shelf life, were not immune, especially since harvest sizes depended on annual fluctuations in weather and other factors. Indeed, the spring was well known as a season prone to food shortages—that risky period at the cusp between the end of last autumn's stores and the beginning of new yields.

In fact, while famine was by no means the norm, the possibility of hunger would have lurked perpetually in the background for many,

and this awareness contributed to a second notable difference: the greater variety of things
considered to be food. The rural poor evidently
had deep knowledge of what kinds of things
could be eaten in a pinch—plants that hovered
on the line between edible and inedible but that
would provide nutrition if all else failed. Indeed,
as a result of natural variation in food availability due to seasonality, combined with farmers'
diversifying precautions against the threat of
crop failure, even the more well-to-do contem-
plated a much wider array of foods than the
typical eater of today. In the selections that follow I have only included foods that will be readily familiar, but the variety of foods discussed
by the authors I draw on is marked. Plants unfamiliar to today's produce section abound, and
the distinctions between what belongs in the
vegetable garden, the ornamental garden, and
the weed pile were quite different in antiquity:
lettuce and turnip find themselves cheek by jowl
with their largely forgotten cousins mallow, or-

ache, sorrel, purslane, alexanders, and cuckoo-pint. This is also true to a lesser extent for the grains. Though wheat and barley were favorites, farmers cultivated a range of varieties and species, like einkorn, emmer, and millet, both to maximize the productivity of their land and to ensure against unforeseen disaster to any one crop (what served as animal fodder in good harvest years could fill the dinner plate as porridge in bad ones). The same flexibility was true of animal products: we hear of milk and eggs from a variety of species and meat derived not just from a wide range of animals but also from all their conceivable parts.

Finally, in the absence of reliable means of refrigeration, the consumption of fresh food tended to be hyperlocal. Local weather and geographical conditions dictated which crops, fruits, and vegetables would grow best in different places and which animals would thrive. Fresh fish was mostly only realistic for those with proximity to places where it could be

caught. Nevertheless, even in the period of the earliest texts considered in this book (the fifth century BCE), there was already a robust trade in foodstuffs, and the variety and geographical reach of food imports grew steadily over the centuries. The three dietary staples—grain, olive oil, and wine—were easily transportable and could be traded across the Mediterranean, especially to serve urban communities that had outgrown their rural hinterlands (the fertile fields of Sicily, Egypt, and North Africa became the breadbaskets of Rome). As networks and wealth increased, so, too, did the variety and availability of different foods from different places, from luxury items for impressive dinner parties to more accessible preserved foods. Salted fish and fish sauce were popular (and comparatively affordable) commodities for import, while the ingenuity of Roman aquaculture surpassed itself in its quest to usher the tastiest fish from their distant homes onto the plates of the superwealthy. Though fans of modern Italian cuisine

will find that neither tomatoes nor pasta had yet arrived, Pliny the Elder records the bonanza of new types of grafted fruits that began flooding the Roman market in the first centuries BCE and CE, joining other exotic fare—like the pistachios from North Africa and Syria, capers from Cyprus, and cane sugar from India and Yemen included in the passages I have collected here. Ancient eaters were aware of the local variations in their food, from both nearer and farther afield. At an extreme level, they took note of the exotic food habits of those on the margins of their own food worlds: consider the passages included in Part II on butter, that strange, barbarian alternative to olive oil. At the more subtle level, they saw variation in quality from place to place, tracking where the best wheat grows, where the best cheeses come from, which fish are best in which places, and other similar local knowledge (the wine snobs of today have nothing on the wine snobs of antiquity).

This increased globalization of the food market, however, led to concerns that may resonate with the modern reader. Though worries about carbon footprints were two millennia in the future, some still felt that it was morally suspect to be eating so many mixed-up things imported from so many mixed-up places. The passage in Part II from the Stoic philosopher Seneca, in which he expresses his skepticism of the casseroles and other compound dishes popular in his time, is characteristic of this viewpoint. More generally, there was a moral backlash against the ostentatious gourmandism that became a popular means of parading wealth in the Roman empire. The moralist Plutarch warns against eating things you have no real appetite for just because they are exotic, and Seneca's strictures against those who "hunt for ways to rouse hunger" rather than to sate it uncannily evoke the modern processed food industry. Food quality was also a concern, especially for urban dwell-

ers. Galen's advice to avoid fish caught at the mouths of contaminated rivers reminds us that pollution is not a uniquely postindustrial problem. The adulteration of shelf-stable items like grain and spices was also a known issue, and various legal and regulatory provisions emerged in an attempt to protect consumers from fraudulent food. More luridly, even centuries before *Sweeney Todd*, there were alarming rumors about the mystery meat served by unscrupulous innkeepers (see the entry on pork in Part II). Finally—though this is likely more distressing to the modern reader than it was to most of the authors collected here—there was enormous variation in quality between the diets of the haves and have-nots. While the rich fretted about gout, bloating, and the other health risks of overindulgence, the poor had to be ready to contend with the perils of sometimes not getting enough. As mentioned above, the rural poor were particularly exposed to the risks inherent

in small-scale farming, where a bad harvest could necessitate inventive food substitutions. The urban poor had even less direct control over their food. Since cooking facilities were a domestic luxury in the city, they had to rely on whatever cookshops were serving for most of their meals, in an ancient twist on the fast-food diet. While this arrangement afforded them a taste of a wider array of ingredients than they would likely have been able to buy for themselves — archaeological analysis of the sewers in Herculaneum has shown that even the comparatively poor had at least a trace of pricey imported pepper in their bellies — it also left the fullness of their stomachs with an uncomfortably direct dependency on the fullness of their purses; many relied to some degree on publicly or privately subsidized food (when they could get it).[3] In short, the ancient advice on dietary choices collected in this book would have been relevant to only that fraction of the ancient population with the luxury to choose.

I conclude this section with what I hope is an obvious disclaimer: this book is not intended to serve as actual dietary or medical advice. For all the commonalities that we may find, ancient Greco-Roman attitudes to food spring from a fundamentally different understanding of the world. Rather, the ancient texts provide us with a way to think about how we think about food. Some of the advice you find here will resonate delightfully with your common sense (if you want to gain weight, eat more fat and sugar!) or your own experience (beans make you flatulent!); some may bewilder you (walking around nude makes you thinner?). On the whole, though, you may find that this encounter with ancient dietetics tends to clarify what is at stake when we think about diet. When we strip away the scientific details, the fundamental issues that underlie dietary choices remain. These ancient voices remind us that humans have long been aware that food is not an independent variable, but rather must be balanced with all other

aspects of a healthy lifestyle; that people have different bodies with different needs; and that being mindful about how your food choices affect your well-being is never a bad idea, whether or not you believe that lettuce is medicinal.

The Texts

The rest of this book is organized in two parts. The first part provides three extended passages that offer dietary and lifestyle advice for the nonspecialist. As the section heading indicates, these passages tell the reader *how* to eat: that is, what sorts of foods to eat, when, and in conjunction with what exercises and other activities. Though a wide range of dietetic literature survives, I chose these specific texts for two reasons. First, they represent three distinct periods in the history of Greco-Roman medical literature and thus offer a survey of dietary thinking: the first text dates to classical Greece of the late fifth century BCE, the second to the Hellenistic world of the mid-fourth century

BCE, and the third to the Roman imperial period of the early first century CE. Second, they are all intended for a general audience; these are not specialized medical diets suited to specific conditions, but broad dietary guidelines to be followed by average, more or less healthy people (average, that is, in medical, not economic terms: as mentioned above, it was only the wealthy minority in the Greco-Roman world who had the time, the resources, the education, and the (literal) freedom to consult books like these and to arrange their days and their diets according to these guidelines). This framing offers two major benefits to today's reader: they are quite easy to understand, even without any explanatory footnotes, and they are engagingly evocative of the normal, everyday choices we make about our food and our bodies. Other texts—those by Galen, for example—go into far greater detail as to why various dietary choices are beneficial in certain cases; while these explanations are fascinating, they are inextricably part and parcel of

contemporary medical views about the body, and therefore deploy terms and concepts that require a significant amount of unpacking for the modern—and, indeed, the ancient—nonspecialist reader. The three dietary regimes provided here, however, were designed to be followed by laypeople. As a result, they are nearly as accessible today as they would have been to their contemporary readers.

The first text, in Greek, is drawn from the Hippocratic *Regimen in Health*. While I have entitled this section "Seasonal Eating with Hippocrates," the "Hippocrates" there is misleading. We do not know what the author of this specific text was named. The fifth century BCE saw a burgeoning of interest in medicine and medical literature in Greece, and a selection of popular medical writings by a variety of authors from this period was later collected and codified under the name of the most famous doctor of the time, Hippocrates. This particular text, which circulated as a part of the larger, more

theoretical text *On the Nature of Man*, offers general dietary advice for the nonmedical reader to follow, beginning with optimal seasonal eating patterns and then adding some specific advice depending on individuals' age, gender, and athleticism. It is a short work, and I reproduce much of it here. I omit only the sections at the end, which digress (contrary to the title) into regimens suitable to various illnesses, and a short passage in the middle on purging. Purging—via both emetics and enemas—was a standard medical tool in antiquity, and some, though by no means all, felt that routine purging was an essential part of a healthy dietary regimen; I felt it too alien to the modern concept of diet to warrant inclusion in the context here.

The second text, also in Greek, is the work of the fourth-century BCE physician Diocles. The fourth century was the beginning of a period of enormous scientific creativity, and dietetics particularly blossomed as a dedicated field of study. Sadly, almost all of the medical

literature from this period has been lost, and Diocles, though a famous and well-reputed doctor in antiquity, was no exception to this rule; thanks to his popularity, however, a significant amount of his work survives embedded as extracts, quotations, or summaries in other authors' writings. We are fortunate that this particularly engaging passage survives at length in a fourth-century CE compendium,[4] and I have reproduced almost the entirety of it here (omitting only a few sentences at the very end, once again on purging). Diocles' advice is personal and almost astonishingly detailed—everything from haircare to timing your bowel movements. As would any good doctor from the period, he locates diet within a nexus of other lifestyle choices: sleeping, bathing, skin care, exercise, sex, and even work responsibilities must all be carefully coordinated with one's food intake and state of digestion. The passage walks the reader through an optimal daily routine, before offer-

ing some brief suggestions for how to adapt it from season to season.

The third and last of these longer texts is the beginning of the first book of Celsus' *On Medicine*. Written in Latin for a general public in the first century CE, this text was a part of Celsus' larger project to provide an encyclopedic survey of the topics he thought a Roman gentleman ought to be familiar with. His basic thesis here is that there is no reason for an intelligent, healthy person to need a doctor to tell him what to eat; rather, a good Roman should be self-sufficient and, merely by reading Celsus' advice and paying attention to what his own body is telling him, should be able to manage his own daily routine for optimal health. Like Diocles, Celsus provides a basic overview of healthy daily habits, first ones suited to robust people and then ones for the more delicate; both sets share an emphasis on self-awareness and flexibility. He then concludes with some

notes for specific situations; here I have taken a more liberal editorial hand than elsewhere, skipping over several paragraphs that were unduly technical or culturally specific.

Part II of this book is a natural sequel to Part I. Once you know the generalities of how to fit dietary choices into your overall lifestyle, the pressing question becomes *what*, specifically, to eat. A range of texts from different genres offer their own answers to this question, and I have drawn on a representative selection in order to reflect the constellation of ideas about food that existed in classical antiquity. Indeed, the most challenging aspect of putting this section together was choosing which foods to include: the literature here is so abundant and the selection of foods eaten in antiquity so varied that I was embarrassed for choice. I have presented a representative array of types of foods; however, rather than attempt to include as many examples of each type as possible, I have chosen only a handful for each, allowing

me space to offer multiple perspectives on many of them. This multiplicity of voices is one of the most delightful things about ancient writing on food: a wide variety of opinions flourished, both evolving from one another and standing happily in contemporaneous tension. Certainly, different authors often agree on some basic commonalities, but there can also be huge variation in the reputations of various foods. Consider lentils, for example: where Roman moralists see a wholesomely simple food, the medical community sees an on-ramp to disease. I hope that the smorgasbord of passages provided will offer a taste of the wild world of food in Greco-Roman antiquity.

It will be helpful to have some background on the various texts to be found here. A large fraction of these passages come from medical sources, the majority from specifically dietetic texts. The longest, most relevant treatise—which accordingly appears most frequently—is Galen's *On the Properties of Foodstuffs*. This text,

written in Greek in the second century CE, systematically describes the effects that individual foods have on the body from a medical perspective; set up almost as an encyclopedia, each food has an individual entry, with a book on grains and legumes, another on fruits and vegetables, and a third on foods derived from animals. A similar, though much more compressed, dietetic list of foods was already circulating in the fifth century BCE and survives today as part of the text in the Hippocratic Corpus known as *Regimen* (not to be confused with the distinct text, *Regimen in Health*, already encountered above). The text as a whole is concerned (like the three passages in Part I) with how diet and digestion fit into the overall picture of health, but it also includes this significant section on the powers of individual foodstuffs, from which I draw several extracts. Outside of dedicated dietetic treatises like these, comments on specific foods also sometimes crop up in more therapeu-

tically or theoretically oriented medical texts, and I have included a few such instances from Galen as well. Further, as we saw above, many plants and animal products were considered as much drug as food; the medical subgenre of pharmaceutical texts therefore often has relevant things to say on our topic. Dioscorides' *Medical Substances* (a Greek text from the first century CE) includes comments about the digestive consequences of some substances when eaten as food, which I have included fairly liberally; these are all imbedded in the broader context of their effects when deployed as drugs (as salves, poultices, ingredients in compound medicines, etc.)—I have occasionally left some of these comments in as well for further color.

Beyond these medical texts, comments on food qualities appear in other genres as well, often to different effect. I have drawn passages from four other genres to round out the picture. The first of these is natural history, which com-

prises topics that today would be siloed into multifarious subfields like botany, zoology, geology, geography, anthropology, and more. Pliny's *Natural History* is an encyclopedic text in Latin in thirty-seven books from the first century CE that includes many chapters related to foods, several of which I have selected here. They tend to have an eclectic feel: the dietary information is mixed up with historical anecdotes, ethnographical observations, and botanical or zoological factoids. The second genre is moral philosophy. Moralists broach the topic of diet with some regularity, due to the overlaps between food consumption, self-control, and decadence. Unsurprisingly, given their different agenda, they often have quite a different spin on foods than the medical authors do. I have included passages from both Seneca's letters and Plutarch's paramedical text, *On Keeping Well*. Seneca (a Roman Stoic philosopher from the first century CE) and Plutarch (a Greek moral

essayist of a Platonist stripe from the late first/
early second century CE) were both demon-
strably familiar with the medical thinking of
their times; however, their opinions about food
are overwhelmingly shaped by their emphasis
on the moral value of a life of self-control and
avoidance of luxuriant indulgences, with the result that their advice can be quite different from
that of their contemporary doctors (for an egre-
gious example, compare Plutarch and Galen on
lentils in Part II). Third is the abundant literature on farming and animal husbandry in antiquity, which often has relevant things to say,
despite coming at foodstuffs from the supplier's
rather than the consumer's perspective. My representative of this genre is Cato's *On Farming*, a
second-century BCE Latin text, which includes
an extensive paean to the cabbage (of which I
have reproduced only a small part!). Finally, we
have one particularly fascinating compendium
from the chef's point of view, namely the late

antique Latin cookbook attached to the name of Apicius, the (in)famous gourmand of the first century CE whose name became synonymous with luxury. I could not resist including a few of its recipes here, ranging from the very familiar (a recipe for honey-glazed ham) to the decidedly foreign (a casserole with everything but the kitchen sink).

A Note on the Translations

In creating the translations provided here, I have attempted to walk the fine line between readability and exactitude. While my English usually conveys both the meaning and the grammar of the original, there are times when adherence to the latter would confuse rather than elucidate the former. Similarly, these texts are often quite lively and informal in their tone, and I have done my best to reproduce that tone, even if it sometimes required a somewhat more liberal construal. The point where I have

most systematically deviated from the original in this regard is in the matter of the verbs in the longer texts that comprise Part I. All three texts offer instructions for diet; however, the grammatical constructions used in each are often impersonal: "one should," "it is fitting to," and so on. But because of the syntax that Greek and Latin employ for these kinds of impersonal constructions, it is often the case that the impersonal subjects are implicit, leaving the verbs standing alone as unmarked infinitives. The overwhelming tenor of these infinitives is instructive, and I have therefore often chosen to render them as imperatives, which come across as more natural and less stilted to the modern reader. In doing so, I introduce a second person singular, or "you," who is not strictly there in the text, though, I think, present in the spirit of the advice. To give a sense of the difference, here is a representative example from each text, translated first literally

and then as I have rendered them in the pages that follow:

Literal translation: Average people ought to arrange their diet in the following way: in the winter [they ought] to eat as much as possible, but to drink as little as possible.

My translation: The average person should arrange their diet in the following way: in the winter, eat as much as possible, but drink as little as possible.

Literal translation: Before dinner, it is fitting to take a walk, empty and retaining no undigested food from earlier meals. One can tell if this is the case . . .

My translation: Before dinner, you ought to walk on an empty stomach that retains no undigested food from earlier meals. You can tell if this is the case . . .

Literal translation: [It is fitting for these sorts of people] to live in a house that is full of light . . . ; to be careful of noonday heat . . . ;

to not expose themselves to weather when
the sun comes in and out in a cloudy sky,
lest now heat, now coldness affect them.

My translation: Advice for these people: live in
a house that is full of light. . . . Be careful of
noonday heat. . . . Don't expose yourself to
weather when the sun comes in and out in a
cloudy sky, which can make you alternatingly hot and cold.

On balance, this approach seemed sufficiently
reflective of the experience of reading the original texts—and sufficiently superior in terms of
engagement and accessibility for readers of the
English—to warrant this slight deviation.

Similarly, I have sometimes chosen to use
terms that will be more readily understand-
able to the modern reader, even if they do not
exactly capture all the nuances of the original
words deployed. Most notably, the topic of
anointing with oil comes up repeatedly in these
texts: the Greeks and Romans often smeared

their bodies with oil, either as part of, or in lieu of, bathing (in which case the dirty oil would be removed) or after bathing (in which case it would be left to soak in). The former practice will be foreign to the day-to-day experience of most readers, but the latter overlaps considerably, in both practice and purpose, with that of moisturizing. I have translated it accordingly wherever suitable, but the reader should imagine more an oily unguent than a modern lotion or cream. Likewise, Celsus speaks of smearing the body with potter's earth, which I translated as having a mud treatment—less specific, but much more recognizable. Such small liberties occur as needed. Finally, the exact identity of some species of plants and animals can be difficult to convey: some species are specific to the Mediterranean and will be unfamiliar to readers from elsewhere, some have evolved or gone extinct, and some are simply unidentifiable from their Greek or Latin names (many a dictionary entry satisfies itself with the woefully

unhelpful "a type of fish"). I have done my best to provide names that accurately convey—or at least evoke—what the author is talking about. The opposite problem can also occur: sometimes the ancient and modern words are the same, but the thing they are referring to would have been subtly (or not so subtly) different. This is true of both disease names and plant names. In the former case, it is the result of our fundamentally different understanding and classification of diseases (the ancient conception of cancer, for instance, should not be mapped directly onto the modern one); in the latter, it is the legacy of two millennia of deliberately manipulative farmers (today's lettuce, for example, is likely a milder and more tender vegetable than the ancestor that Galen was using as a drug—though he would no doubt be gratified to learn that lettuce water is nevertheless back in vogue as an Internet sensation for curing insomnia!).

PART I

How to Eat

Hippocratic *Regimen in Health* 1–4, 6–7

[1] τοὺς ἰδιώτας ὧδε χρὴ διαιτᾶσθαι· τοῦ μὲν χειμῶνος ἐσθίειν ὡς πλεῖστα, πίνειν δὲ ὡς ἐλάχιστα·
εἶναι δὲ χρὴ τὸ πόμα οἶνον ὡς ἀκρητέστατον, τὰ
δὲ σιτία ἄρτον καὶ τὰ ὄψα ὀπτὰ πάντα, λαχάνοισι
δὲ ὡς ἐλαχίστοισι χρῆσθαι ταύτην τὴν ὥρην·
οὕτω γὰρ ἂν μάλιστα τὸ σῶμα ξηρόν τε εἴη καὶ

SEASONAL EATING WITH HIPPOCRATES

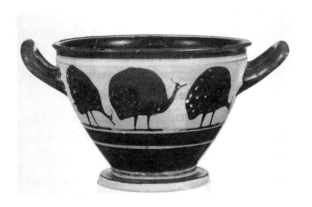

[1] The average person should arrange their diet in the following way: in the winter, eat as much as possible, but drink as little as possible. Drink should be wine as undiluted as possible, and food should be bread and dishes prepared exclusively by roasting; eat as few vegetables as

θερμόν. ὅταν δὲ τὸ ἔαρ ἐπιλαμβάνῃ, τό τε πόμα χρὴ πλέον ποιεῖσθαι καὶ ὑδαρέστερον καὶ κατ᾽ ὀλίγον, καὶ τοῖσι σιτίοισι μαλακωτέροισι χρῆσθαι καὶ ἐλάσσοσι καὶ τῶν ἄρτων ἀφαιρέοντα μάζαν προστιθέναι καὶ τὰ ὄψα κατὰ τὸν αὐτὸν λόγον ἐκ τῶν ὀπτῶν ἑφθὰ ποιεῖσθαι καὶ λαχάνοισιν ἤδη χρῆσθαι τοῦ ἦρος ὀλίγοισιν, ὅπως ἐς τὴν θερείην καταστήσεται ὥνθρωπος τοῖσί τε σιτίοισι μαλθα-κοῖσι πᾶσι χρεώμενος καὶ τοῖσιν ὄψοισιν ἑφθοῖσι καὶ λαχάνοισιν ὠμοῖσι καὶ ἑφθοῖσι καὶ τοῖσι πόμα-σιν ὡς ὑδαρεστάτοισι καὶ πλείστοισι, καὶ μὴ με-γάλη ἡ μεταβολὴ ἔσται ἐξαπίνης χρεωμένῳ τοῦ [δὲ] θέρεος τῇ τε μάζῃ μαλθακῇ καὶ τῷ πόματι ὑδαρεῖ καὶ πολλῷ καὶ τοῖσιν ὄψοισιν ἑφθοῖσι πᾶσι· δεῖ γὰρ χρῆσθαι τούτοισιν, ὅταν τὸ θέρος ᾖ, ὅπως τὸ σῶμα ψυχρὸν καὶ μαλθακὸν γένηται· ἡ γὰρ ὥρη θερμή τε καὶ ξηρή, καὶ παρέχεται τὰ σώματα καυματώδεα καὶ αὐχμηρά· δεῖ οὖν τοῖσιν ἐπιτη-δεύμασιν ἀλέξασθαι. κατὰ δὲ τὸν αὐτὸν λόγον, ὥσπερ ἐν τῷ ἦρι ἐκ τοῦ χειμῶνος ἐς τὸ θέρος κα-ταστῆσαι τῶν μὲν σιτίων ἀφαιρέοντα, τῷ δὲ ποτῷ προστιθέντα, οὕτω δὲ καὶ τὰ ἐναντία ποιέοντα

possible in this season. For in this way the body will be as dry and warm as possible. But whenever spring approaches, it is necessary to make your drinks more abundant and more diluted and to sip at them frequently; also to partake of softer food and less of it: cut down on breads and replace them with barley cakes; by the same logic, make your dishes stewed instead of roasted; already in the spring a person can incorporate a few vegetables, so that as it comes to be summer they are eating all soft foods (stewed main dishes and raw and stewed vegetables) and drinks as diluted and copious as possible. It should not be a sudden, drastic change to the summer regime of soft barley cakes and frequent, diluted drinks and only dishes that are stewed. It is necessary to partake of these sorts of things whenever it is hot, so that the body can be cool and soft; for the season is hot and dry and renders bodies burning and parched, making it necessary to avert this outcome by means of these habits. Just as in

καταστῆσαι ἐκ τοῦ θέρεος ἐς τὸν χειμῶνα ἐν [δὲ] τῷ φθινοπώρῳ, τὰ μὲν σιτία πλείω ποιεύμενον καὶ ξηρότερα καὶ τὰ ὄψα κατὰ λόγον, τὰ δὲ ποτὰ ἐλάσσω καὶ ἀκρητέστερα, ὅπως ὅ τε χειμὼν ἀγαθὸς ἔσται καὶ ὤνθρωπος διαχρήσεται τοῖσί τε πόμασιν ἀκρητεστάτοισιν καὶ ὀλίγοισι καὶ τοῖσι σιτίοισι ὡς πλείστοισί τε καὶ ξηροτάτοισι· οὕτω γὰρ ἂν καὶ ὑγιαίνοι μάλιστα καὶ ῥιγῴη ἥκιστα· ἡ γὰρ ὥρη ψυχρή τε καὶ ὑγρή.

[2] τοῖσι δὲ εἴδεσι τοῖσι σαρκώδεσι καὶ μαλθακοῖσι καὶ ἐρυθροῖσι συμφέρει τὸν πλείω χρόνον τοῦ ἐνιαυτοῦ ξηροτέροισι τοῖσι διαιτήμασι χρῆσθαι· ὑγρὴ γὰρ ἡ φύσις τῶν εἰδέων τούτων. τοὺς δὲ στιφροὺς καὶ προσεσταλμένους καὶ πυρροὺς καὶ μέλανας τῇ ὑγροτέρῃ διαίτῃ χρῆσθαι τὸν πλείω χρόνον· τὰ γὰρ σώματα ταῦτα ὑπάρχει ξηρὰ ἐόντα. καὶ τοῖσι νέοισι τῶν σωμάτων συμφέρει μαλθακωτέροισι καὶ ὑγροτέροισι χρῆσθαι

the spring you transitioned from winter into summer by cutting down on food and ramping up on drinks, you should apply the same logic also to the transition from summer into winter by doing the opposite in the autumn: eating more food (and drier) and dealing with dishes appropriately, and as for drinks, making them less copious and less diluted, so that when it is good and winter, you will be habituated to infrequent drinks, very little diluted, and food that is as abundant and dry as possible. For in this way one will be most healthy and least shivery, for the season is cold and wet.

[2] For those whose constitutions are fleshy, soft, and ruddy: it is advantageous to use a drier diet for the majority of the year since the nature of these sorts of constitutions is moist. But people who are firm-bodied, lean, and red- or black-haired ought to use a moister diet most of the time since those bodies tend to be dry. For younger bodies, it is advantageous to use softer and moister diets since their time of life is dry

τοῖσι διαιτήμασι· ἡ γὰρ ἡλικίη ξηρή, καὶ τὰ σώματα πέπηγεν ἔτι· τοὺς δὲ πρεσβυτέρους τῷ ξηροτέρῳ τρόπῳ χρὴ τὸ πλέον τοῦ χρόνου διάγειν·
τὰ γὰρ σώματα ἐν ταύτῃ τῇ ἡλικίῃ ὑγρὰ καὶ μαλ-
θακὰ καὶ ψυχρά. δεῖ οὖν πρὸς τὴν ἡλικίην καὶ τὴν
ὥρην καὶ τὰ εἴδεα τὰ διαιτήματα ποιεῖσθαι ἐν-
αντιούμενον τοῖσι καθισταμένοισι καὶ θάλπεσι καὶ
χειμῶσιν· οὕτω γὰρ ἂν μάλιστα ὑγιαίνοιεν.

[3] καὶ ὁδοιπορεῖν τοῦ μὲν χειμῶνος ταχέως
χρή, τοῦ δὲ θέρεος ἡσυχῇ, ἢν μὴ δι᾽ ἡλίου ὁδοι-
πορῇ· δεῖ δὲ τοὺς μὲν σαρκώδεας θᾶσσον ὁδοιπορεῖν, τοὺς δὲ ἰσχνοὺς ἡσυχέστερον. λουτροῖσι
δὲ χρὴ πολλοῖσι χρῆσθαι τοῦ θέρεος, τοῦ δὲ χειμῶνος ἐλάσσοσι· τοὺς στιφροὺς χρὴ μᾶλλον
λούεσθαι τῶν σαρκωδέων. ἠμφιέσθαι δὲ χρὴ
τοῦ μὲν χειμῶνος καθαρὰ ἱμάτια, τοῦ δὲ θέρεος
ἐλαιοπινέα.

[4] τοὺς παχέας χρή, ὅσοι βούλονται λεπτοὶ
γενέσθαι, τὰς ταλαιπωρίας νήστιας ἐόντας
ποιεῖσθαι ἁπάσας, καὶ τοῖσι σιτίοισιν ἐπιχειρεῖν
ἀσθμαίνοντας καὶ μὴ ἀνεψυγμένους καὶ προπε-

and their bodies are still solid. But more elderly people ought to use a drier diet most of the time, since bodies at that time of life are moist, soft, and cold. In sum, it is necessary to plan people's diets in accordance with age and season and constitutions, opposing the prevailing conditions, whether hot or cold. For in this way one will be healthiest.

[3] Further, it is necessary to walk briskly in the winter, but to stroll in the summer (as long as you are not walking in the sun). Those who are fleshy should walk more briskly, those who are scrawny more slowly. It is necessary to take many baths in the summer, fewer in the winter; and the firm-bodied ought to bathe more frequently than the fleshy. In the winter it is necessary to wear washed garments, but in the summer they should be treated with oil.

[4] Any stout people who wish to become thin should do all exercise in a state of fasting; they should take their meals while breathing hard and not yet having cooled down, and they

πωκότας οἶνον κεκρημένον μὴ σφόδρα ψυχρόν·
καὶ τὰ ὄψα σκευάζειν σησάμοισιν ἡδύσμασι καὶ
τοῖσι ἄλλοισι τοῖσι τοιουτοτρόποισι· καὶ πίονα δὲ
ἔστω· οὕτω γὰρ ἂν ἀπὸ ἐλαχίστων ἐμπιπλαῖντο·
καὶ μονοσιτεῖν καὶ ἀλουτεῖν καὶ σκληροκοιτεῖν
καὶ γυμνὸν περιπατεῖν ὅσον οἷόν τε μάλιστ᾽ ἂν ᾖ.
ὅσοι δὲ βούλονται λεπτοὶ ἐόντες παχεῖς γενέσθαι, τά τε ἄλλα ποιεῖν τἀναντία κείνοισι, καὶ νήστιας μηδεμίαν ταλαιπωρίην ποιεῖσθαι. . . .

[6] τὰ δὲ παιδία χρὴ τὰ νήπια βρέχειν ἐν θερμῷ
ὕδατι πολλὸν χρόνον, καὶ πίνειν διδόναι ὑδαρέα
τὸν οἶνον καὶ μὴ ψυχρὸν παντάπασι, τοῦτον δὲ
διδόναι, ὃς ἥκιστα τὴν γαστέρα μετεωριεῖ καὶ
φῦσαν παρέξει· ταῦτα δὲ ποιεῖν, ὅπως οἵ τε σπα-
σμοὶ ἧσσον ἐπιλαμβάνωσιν, καὶ μέζονα γίνηται
καὶ εὐχροώτερα. τὰς γυναῖκας χρὴ διαιτᾶσθαι τῷ
ξηροτέρῳ τῶν τρόπων· καὶ γὰρ τὰ σιτία ξηρὰ ἐπι-
τηδειότερα πρὸς τὴν μαλθακότητα τῶν σαρκῶν,

should drink diluted, not very cold wine before they eat. They should prepare their dishes with sesame sauce and other similar sorts of seasonings, and these dishes should be high in fat so that they feel satiated after the smallest amount. Further, they should take only one meal a day, avoid bathing, sleep on a firm mattress, and walk around in the nude as often as possible. Any thin people who wish to bulk up should do the exact opposite of these things, and never exert themselves while fasting. . . .

[6] Infant children should be given long, warm baths and should be given watered-down wine to drink,[1] which is not completely cold; they should be given a wine least likely to unsettle their stomach or cause gas. We do these things so that they are less likely to have convulsions and so that they grow bigger and rosier-cheeked. Women ought to follow a comparatively dry diet, since dry foods are better suited to the softness of their flesh, and less

καὶ τὰ πόματα ἀκρητέστερα ἀμείνω πρὸς τὰς ὑστέρας καὶ τὰς κυοτροφίας.

[7] τοὺς γυμναζομένους χρὴ τοῦ χειμῶνος καὶ τρέχειν καὶ παλαίειν, τοῦ δὲ θέρεος παλαίειν μὲν ὀλίγα, τρέχειν δὲ μή, περιπατεῖν δὲ πολλὰ κατὰ ψῦχος. ὅσοι κοπιῶσιν ἐκ τῶν δρόμων, τούτους παλαίειν χρή· ὅσοι δ᾽ ἂν παλαίοντες κοπιῶσιν, τούτους τρέχειν χρή· οὕτω γὰρ ἂν ταλαιπωρέοντι τὸ κοπιῶν τοῦ σώματος διαθερμαίνοιτο καὶ διαναπαύοιτο μάλιστα. ὁπόσους μάλιστα γυμναζομένους διάρροιαι λαμβάνουσι, καὶ τὰ ὑποχωρήματα σιτώδεα καὶ ἄπεπτα, τούτοισι τῶν τε γυμνασίων ἀφαιρεῖν μὴ ἐλάσσω τοῦ τρίτου μέρεος, καὶ τῶν σιτίων τοῖσιν ἡμίσεσιν χρῆσθαι· δῆλον γὰρ δὴ ὅτι ἡ κοιλίη συνθάλπειν οὐ δύναται ὥστε πέσσεσθαι τὸ πλῆθος τῶν ἐσιόντων σιτίων· ἔστω δὲ τούτοισι τὰ σιτία ἄρτος ἐξοπτότατος, ἐν οἴνῳ ἐντεθρυμμένος, καὶ τὰ ποτὰ ἀκρητέστατα καὶ ἐλάχιστα, καὶ περιπάτοισι μὴ χρήσθωσαν ἀπὸ τοῦ σιτίου· μονοσιτεῖν δὲ χρὴ ὑπὸ τοῦτον τὸν χρόνον· οὕτω γὰρ ἂν μάλιστα συνθάλποιτο ἡ κοιλίη, καὶ τῶν ἐσιόντων ἐπικρατέοι. γίνεται δὲ ὁ τρόπος οὗτος

diluted drinks are better for the womb and for childbearing.

[7] People who exercise ought to both run and wrestle during the winter, but in the summer, they should wrestle infrequently and cease to run, and instead walk about a lot when it is cool. Any of them who have grown sore from running ought to switch to wrestling, while those who are sore from wrestling should run: exerting themselves in this way will warm and rest the sore part of the body optimally. People who find themselves seized with diarrhea after intensive exercise and have stool full of undigested food ought to ramp down their exercise to no less than a third of what it was and to consume half as much food. For it is obvious that their stomach is not able to reach a level of heat adequate to digest the quantity of food that was eaten. They should eat very well-baked bread crumbled up in wine, their drinks should be very little diluted and as infrequent as possible, and they should not take walks after meals.

τῆς διαρροίης τῶν σωμάτων τοῖσι πυκνοσάρ-
κοισι μάλιστα, ὅταν ἀναγκάζηται ὥνθρωπος κρεη-
φαγεῖν, τῆς φύσιος ὑπαρχούσης τοιαύτης· αἱ γὰρ
φλέβες πυκνωθεῖσαι οὐκ ἀντιλαμβάνονται τῶν
σιτίων τῶν ἐσιόντων· ἔστιν δὲ αὕτη μὲν ἡ φύσις
ὀξέα, καὶ τρέπεται ἐφ᾽ ἑκάτερα, καὶ ἀκμάζει ὀλίγον χρόνον ἡ εὐεξίη ἐν τοῖσι τοιουτοτρόποισι
τῶν σωμάτων. τὰ δὲ ἀραιότερα τῶν εἰδέων καὶ
δασύτερα καὶ τὴν ἀναγκοφαγίην δέχεται, καὶ τὰς
ταλαιπωρίας μάλιστα, καὶ χρονιώτεραι γίνονται
αὐτοῖσιν αἱ εὐεξίαι. . . .

They should take one meal a day during this period. For in this way the stomach will heat up most efficiently and prevail over what is eaten. This type of diarrhea occurs most often in people with densely fleshed bodies, whenever a person naturally of that sort of constitution is forced to eat meat; for their veins, being constricted, do not lay hold of the ingested food. This sort of nature exists on a razor's edge: it can change in either direction, and good health is at its prime for only a short time in these sorts of bodies. The more slender and hairier types of constitution are receptive to lack of choice in their food and to extreme exertion; the peak of their good health is of longer duration. . . .

LIFESTYLE MANAGEMENT
WITH DIOCLES

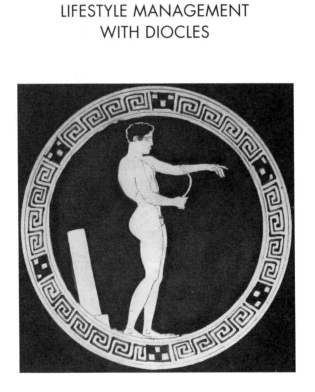

Diocles, *Regimen for Health* (Fragment 182)

[1] ἀρχὴ μέν ἐστι τῆς τῶν ὑγιεινῶν πραγματείας ἡ ἐκ τῶν ὕπνων εἰς τὸ ἐγρηγορέναι μετάβασις· ἐγείρεσθαι δ᾽ ὡς ἐπὶ τὸ πολὺ καλῶς ἔχει μεθεστη- κότων ἤδη τῶν σιτίων ἐκ τῆς ἄνω γαστρὸς ἐπὶ τὴν κάτω κοιλίαν. καλῶς δ᾽ ἔχει τὸν νέον καὶ ἀκ- μάζοντα μικρὸν πρὸ ἡλίου ὅσον διελθεῖν στάδια δέκα, θέρους δ᾽ ὅσον πέντε, τὸν δὲ πρεσβύτερον ἐλάσσω τούτων καὶ θέρους καὶ χειμῶνος. διυπνι- σθέντα δὲ μὴ εὐθὺς ἀνίστασθαι, μένειν δ᾽ ἕως ἂν τὸ δυσκίνητον καὶ νωχελὲς τὸ ἐκ τῶν ὕπνων γινό- μενον ἐκλείπῃ.

[2] μετὰ δὲ τὴν ἀνάστασιν ἁρμόττει πρὸς τοὺς τραχηλισμοὺς τοὺς ὑπὸ τῶν προσκεφαλαίων γι- νομένους ἀνατρίβεσθαι τὸν τράχηλον καὶ τὴν κε- φαλὴν εὖ καὶ καλῶς· ἔπειτα τοῖς μὲν μὴ εὐθὺς εἰθισμένοις κενοῦσθαι τὴν κοιλίαν, καὶ πρὶν κενω- θῆναι, τοῖς δ᾽ ὅταν κενωθῶσιν, εὐθὺς πρὸ τοῦ πράττειν ἄλλο τι, βέλτιόν ἐστιν ἤδη τρίβεσθαι τὸ

[1] The first step in a practical approach to health lies in the transition from sleep to awakening. Things are going well when awakening occurs, for the most part, after the food has already moved from the stomach above to the bowels below. It is a good idea for the young and those in the prime of life to wake up a little before dawn—about twenty minutes, ten in the summer—for older people, a little closer to dawn than this, both in summer and in winter. When you wake up, you should not immediately arise, but remain lying down until the sleep-induced stiffness and sluggishness have ceased.

[2] After getting up, it is suitable to massage your neck and head thoroughly to address any stiffness that has arisen from lying on the pillow. Then, before voiding your bowels (at least, for those accustomed to not immediately doing so; after having done so, for those who are), it is best to immediately—before doing anything

σῶμα πᾶν μετ᾽ ἐλαίου μικροῦ, τοῦ μὲν θέρους
ὕδατος μιγνυμένου, τοῦ δὲ χειμῶνος ὡς ἔχει, χρόνον μὴ ὀλίγον, καὶ μαλακῶς δὲ καὶ ὁμαλῶς, τὸ
ὅλον ἐκτείνοντα καὶ συγκάμπτοντα καὶ πολλάκις
πάντα τὰ ἐνδεχόμενα τοῦ σώματος· ἄμεινον γὰρ
<ἄν> τις καὶ πρὸς ὑγίειαν καὶ πρὸς πάντα πόνον
οὕτως εἴη διακείμενος. μετὰ δὲ ταῦτα τὸ μὲν πρό-
σωπον καὶ τοὺς ὀφθαλμοὺς ὕδατι ψυχρῷ καὶ κα-
θαρῷ προσκλύζειν καὶ ἀπονίζειν καθ᾽ ἑκάστην
ἡμέραν καθαραῖς ταῖς χερσί, τὰ δ᾽ οὖλα πρὸς τοὺς
ὀδόντας [δὲ] καὶ τοὺς ὀδόντας ἢ οὕτως [ἂν] τοῖς
δακτύλοις αὐτοῖς <ἢ> γλήχωνος τετριμμένης ὁμοῦ
λείας παρατρίβειν, καὶ ἐντὸς καὶ ἐκτός, καὶ ἀπο-
σμᾶν τὰ προσκαθήμενα αὐτοῖς ἀπὸ τῶν σιτίων,
τὴν δὲ ῥῖνα καὶ τὰ ὦτα διαχρίειν μὲν καὶ λιπαί-
νειν ἔσωθεν ἀμφότερα, μάλιστα μὲν μύρῳ ἡδεῖ,
εἰ δὲ μή, ἐλαίῳ ὡς ὅτι καθαρωτάτῳ καὶ εὐωδε-
στάτῳ, καὶ ἔσωθεν καὶ ἔξωθεν ἀλείφειν [καὶ]
ταῖς χερσὶ πλατείαις. οὐχ ἥκιστα δὲ τῆς κεφαλῆς
ἐπιμελεῖσθαι δεῖ· θεραπεία δὲ κεφαλῆς ἐστιν, ὡς
οὕτως εἰπεῖν, τρῖψις καὶ χρῖσις καὶ σμῆξις καὶ κτενισμὸς καὶ ἐν χρῷ κουρά. δεῖ δὲ τρίβειν μὲν καὶ

else!—rub down the entire body with a little bit
of olive oil. In the summer, mix it with water;
in the winter, use it straight. Don't rush, and rub
it in gently and evenly, smoothing it all in, bending around, and getting all possible parts of the
body repeatedly. Proceeding in this way will set
you up better both for health and for all types
of exertion. When that is done, splash your face
and eyes with cold, clean water and wash them
off every day with clean hands. Then brush
your teeth and the gums around your teeth,
either with just your fingers or with pennyroyal[1] kneaded into a smooth paste; get both
the inside and the outside and wipe them clean
of anything that has stuck to them from your
food. As to your nose and ears, moisturize them
(making sure to get inside both), preferably with
a sweet unguent, otherwise with olive oil as pure
and pleasant smelling as possible; anoint them
both inside and outside with the flats of your
hands. Your head should receive no small share
of your attention! The way to take care of your

ἀλείφειν αὐτὴν καθ᾽ ἑκάστην ἡμέραν, σμᾶν δὲ καὶ κτενίζειν διά τινων χρόνων. ποιεῖ δ᾽ ἡ μὲν τρῖψις τὸ δερμάτιον ἰσχυρότερον, ἡ δὲ χρῖσις μαλακώτερον, ἡ δὲ σμῆξις τοὺς πόρους καθαρωτέρους καὶ εὐπνοωτέρους, ὁ δὲ κτενισμὸς ἀναξύων καὶ ὁμαλὸν ποιῶν τὸ περὶ τὰς τρίχας ἐκκαθαίρει καὶ περιαιρεῖ τὰ ἐνοχλοῦντα.

[3] μετὰ δὲ τὴν εἰρημένην ἐκ τῶν ὕπνων ἐπιμέλειαν τοὺς μὲν ἕτερόν τι πράττειν ἀναγκαζομένους ἢ προαιρουμένους ἐπὶ τοῦτο ὑποχωρεῖν εὖ ἔχει, τοὺς δὲ σχολάζοντας προπεριπατεῖν ἁρμόζει τὸ σύμμετρον τῇ ῥώμῃ τῆς δυνάμεως. οἱ μὲν οὖν πρὸ τῆς προσφορᾶς τῶν σιτίων πλείους γινόμενοι, κενοῦντες τὸ σῶμα, δεκτικωτέρους τῆς τροφῆς καὶ πέττειν τὰ βρωθέντα ποιοῦσι δυνατωτέρους· οἱ δ᾽ ἀπὸ τῶν σιτίων μέτριοι μὲν ὄντες καὶ βραδεῖς ὁμαλίζουσί τε καὶ μιγνύουσι τὰ σιτία καὶ τὸ ποτὸν καὶ τὰ συγκαταλαμβανόμενα τῶν πνευμάτων αὐτοῖς καὶ τὰ πρόχειρα τῶν περιττωμάτων

head, to put it neatly, is: massage, moisturizing, cleansing, combing, and close shaves. You have to massage and anoint it every day, and wash and comb it periodically. Massage makes your skin stronger, while moisturizing makes it softer; washing makes the pores cleaner and less clogged, and combing, by scraping things down and making everything about the hair even, tidies up and removes any tangles.

[3] After the postsleep routine just described, for those who are obliged (or choose) to do some other business, this is a good time for them to head off to that. For those who have the time, it is suitable to begin with a walk, going as briskly as their strength allows. Longer walks taken before eating meals, by emptying the body, make people more receptive of their food and more able to digest what they have eaten. Walks after meals, provided they are moderate in length and slow, mix together and amalgamate the food and drink (and whatever air got

ἐκκρίνοντες λαπάττουσιν, εὐογκότερον ποιοῦν-
τες τὸν ὄγκον τοῦ πληρώματος, ἀπό τε τῶν
ὑποχονδρίων καταβιβάζοντες τὰς περὶ τὴν κεφαλὴν αἰσθήσεις βελτίους ποιοῦσι καὶ τοὺς ὕπνους
ἀταρακτοτέρους· τοὺς δὲ πολλοὺς καὶ ταχεῖς τῶν
μετὰ τὰ σιτία πρὸς οὐδὲν ἄν τις ἐπαινέσειεν· σεί-
οντες γὰρ ἰσχυρῶς τὸ σῶμα διακρίνουσί τε καὶ
χωρίζουσιν ἀπ᾽ ἀλλήλων τὰ σιτία καὶ τὰ ποτά,
ὥστε κλύδαξίν τε γίνεσθαι καὶ δυσπεψίαν καὶ
τὴν κοιλίαν ἐπιταράττεσθαι πολλάκις.

[4] συμφέρει δὲ μετὰ τὸν περίπατον καθεζόμε-
νον οἰκονομεῖν τι τῶν καθ᾽ αὑτὸν ἕκαστον, ἕως
ἂν ὥρα γένηται τραπέσθαι πρὸς τὴν τοῦ σώματος
ἐπιμέλειαν. καλῶς δ᾽ ἔχει γυμνάζεσθαι τοὺς μὲν
νέους καὶ πλειόνων γυμνασίων γλιχομένους καὶ
δεομένους εἰς τὸ γυμνάσιον ἀποχωρήσαντας,
τοὺς δὲ πρεσβυτέρους καὶ ἀσθενεστέρους εἰς βα-
λανεῖον ἢ εἰς ἄλλην ἀλέαν χρίεσθαι. ἀπόχρη δὲ
τοῖς τηλικούτοις καὶ παντάπασιν ἰδιωτικὸν ἔχου-
σιν αὐτοῖς γυμνάσιον τρῖψις μετρία καὶ μικρὰ κί-
νησις τοῦ σώματος. τρίβεσθαι δὲ βέλτιόν ἐστι τὸν

taken in with them) and empty out any residues that are ready to be expelled, making the burden of a full belly more compact; by drawing down this burden away from the diaphragm, they also improve perception in the head and make sleep less disturbed. But no one would recommend lengthy, brisk walks after meals. For, by roughly shaking up the body, they separate and divide the food and drink from each other, causing gurgling and poor digestion and often disturbing the bowels.

[4] After your walk is a suitable time to sit down and take care of whatever household business you have to do until the hour arrives to turn to taking care of your body. It is a good idea for young people (both those who are really into exercise and those who require it) to retire to a gym and do gymnastic exercise; older and weaker people should go to a bath house instead or anoint themselves in some other warm location. A moderate massage and some gentle movement of the body is sufficient for people

τρίψεως δεόμενον μήτε κεχρισμένον πολὺ μήτε ξηρὸν παντελῶς, ἀλλ᾽ ὑπαλειψάμενον καὶ τριψάμενον ὁμαλῶς, ἔπειτα περιξυσάμενον λουτρῷ ἁρμόττοντι χρήσασθαι, τοὺς δ᾽ ἀσθενεῖς καὶ σφόδρα πρεσβύτας ἀλείφεσθαι [μὲν] λιπαρῶς καὶ ὁμαλῶς. τρίβεσθαι δ᾽ αὐτὸν ὑφ᾽ ἑαυτοῦ τὰ πλεῖστα βέλτιόν ἐστιν· ἅμα γὰρ τῇ τρίψει καὶ γυμνάζεσθαι τὸ σῶμα συμβαίνει δι᾽ ἑαυτοῦ κινούμενον· τὸ δ᾽ ὑφ᾽ ἑτέρου τρίβεσθαι διὰ παντὸς τοῖς κοπιῶσι καὶ τοῖς ἀσθενεστέροις καὶ ῥαθυμοτέρως ἔχουσι πρὸς τὰ γυμνάσια δεῖ μάλιστα ἀπονέμειν.

[5] μετὰ δὲ τὴν θεραπείαν τοῦ σώματος ἐπ᾽ ἄριστον ἀποχωρεῖν· οὐκ ἄδηλον δ᾽ ὅτι καὶ τὸ ἄριστον καὶ πᾶσαν ἁπλῶς τὴν δίαιταν ἁρμόσει τοῦ μὲν θέρους εἶναι μὴ θερμαντικὴν μηδὲ ξηραντικήν, τοῦ δὲ χειμῶνος μήτε ψυκτικὴν μήτε ὑγραντικήν, τοῦ δ᾽ ἔαρος καὶ τοῦ μετοπώρου μέσον τι

of that age and, really, for everyone who has their own private gym. Those who require a massage should receive one without being excessively covered in massage oil, but also not left completely dry. They should be anointed and massaged uniformly, and then scrape themselves clean and avail themselves of a pleasantly warm bath.[2] But the ailing and very elderly should skip the bath and instead be anointed uniformly with a greasy substance. For the most part, it is better to massage yourself; for in that way, you also contrive to exercise your body by moving it around during the massage. But it is very important to ensure massage by someone else for people who are sore or just kind of weak or lazy when it comes to exercise.

[5] After this care of the body, go to lunch. And it is obvious that both lunch and one's entire diet in general should not be warming and drying in the summer and not be cooling and moistening in the winter and should be a happy medium in the spring and the autumn. For those

ἔχουσαν. τοῖς μὲν οὖν εὐόγκως βουλομένοις διά-
γειν τοῦ θέρους ἄριστον ἀποχρῶν ἐστι καὶ πρὸς
ὑγίειαν καὶ πρὸς τὸ διημερεύειν ἱκανῶς ἄλφιτον
λευκὸν χρήσιμον μέτριον ἐπ᾽ οἴνῳ λευκῷ εὐώδει
καὶ μέλιτι μὴ πολλῷ καὶ ὕδατι κεκραμένοις καλῶς
πινόμενον ἢ ἕψημά τι τῶν ἀφύσων καὶ εὐπέπτων
καὶ τροφίμων, καὶ οὕτως καὶ μετὰ μικροῦ μέλιτος
λαμβανόμενον μὴ θερμόν. τῷ δὲ μηδὲν προσιε-
μένῳ τοιοῦτον ἄρτον ἀριστᾶν ἁρμόττει ψυχρὸν
τοσοῦτον ὅσον ἔσται πρὸ τοῦ δειλινοῦ γυμνασίου
καταπέψαι δυνατός. ὄψον δ᾽ ἕξει λάχανον ἑφθὸν
ἢ κολοκύντην ἢ σίκυον ἢ ἄλλο τι τῶν πρὸς τὴν
παροῦσαν ὥραν μὴ ἀναρμόστων ἡψημένον
ἁπλῶς. πίνειν δὲ λευκὸν οἶνον ὑδαρέστερον ἄχρι
τοῦ μὴ διψῆσαι. πρὸ δὲ τοῦ λαμβάνειν τὸ σιτίον
προπίνειν ὕδωρ μέν, ἂν διψᾷ τις, πλεῖον, εἰ δὲ μή,
ἔλαττον.

[6] μετὰ δὲ τὸ ἄριστον μὴ πολὺν διατρίψαντα
χρόνον καταδαρθεῖν ἐν σκοτεινῷ ἢ ψυχεινῷ τόπῳ

who wish to pass their summer at a moderate weight, it is best to content yourself—both for a balance of health and for sufficient sustenance to last the day—with drinking a serviceably moderate amount of white barley that you have mixed up well into sweet-smelling white wine and a little honey and water; or else any kind of porridge of easily-digestible, non-flatulent, nourishing stuff, whether straight or with a little bit of honey (but be sure not to eat it hot). Someone who refuses to eat this quasi-bread will do best to eat any cold lunch that can be digested before the afternoon's exercise. As a main dish, you will have a stewed vegetable, either squash or cucumber or anything else in season that is not ill-suited to being boiled in a simple way. Drink rather diluted white wine, just enough so that you are not thirsty. Before you eat your food, drink some water: more if you're thirsty, less if you're not.

[6] After lunch, don't let much time pass before you take a nap in a shady or cool place, free

καὶ χωρὶς πνεύματος· ἐγερθέντος δέ, οἰκονομεῖν τι τῶν ἰδίων καὶ περιπατεῖν, περιπατήσαντα δὲ καὶ μικρὰ προδιαναπαύσαντα πρὸς τὸ γυμνάσιον ἀποχωρεῖν. καὶ τοῖς μὲν ἰσχυροτέροις καὶ νεωτέροις γυμνασαμένους καὶ κονισαμένους τῷ ψυχρῷ λούεσθαι καλῶς ἔχει· τοὺς δὲ πρεσβυτέρους καὶ ἀσθενεστέρους ἀλειψαμένους καὶ μικρὰ τριψαμένους λούεσθαι θερμῷ, τὴν κεφαλὴν μὴ βρέχοντας. ὁμοίως δὲ πᾶσι τοῖς ὑγιαίνουσι θερμῷ λούσασθαι τὴν κεφαλὴν ὀλιγάκις ἢ οὐδέποτε ἁρμόττει· τοῖς δὲ πρεσβυτέροις οὐδὲ βρέχειν πολλάκις βέλτιόν ἐστιν, ἀλλὰ διά τινων χρόνων χρίεσθαι τῷ ἐλαίῳ, μίσγοντας τοῦ μὲν θέρους ὕδωρ, τοῦ δὲ χειμῶνος οἶνον. ὡς μέγιστον δὲ καὶ βέλτιστον καὶ ἀλειψαμένους ἐκμάττεσθαι καθαρῶς ἢ ἀποσμᾶσθαι καὶ ψυχρῷ μετρίως ἐκκλύζεσθαι καὶ μετὰ τὸ ὑγρᾶναι ἀλείφεσθαι.

[7] πρὸς δὲ τὰ σιτία δεῖ βαδίζειν κενοὺς καὶ μηδὲν ἄπεπτον ἔχοντας τῶν βρωθέντων πρότερον· γινώσκοι δ᾽ ἄν τις τοῦτο μάλιστα τῇ τῶν

from drafts. When you wake up, do some household business and take a stroll; once you've had a stroll and a bit of a rest, retire to the gym. For stronger and younger people, it is a good idea to do some gymnastic exercise covered in dust and then take a cold bath; older and weaker people should give themselves a small massage with oil and then take a warm bath, without getting their head wet. Likewise, it is suitable for all healthy people to wash their head in warm water only infrequently or never. It is better for older people not to get it wet often, but instead to periodically anoint it with oil, mixing in water in the summer, and wine in the winter. It is supremely important and advantageous, once you have anointed yourself, to sponge or wipe yourself clean and rinse in moderately cold water and then moisturize after you've gotten wet.

[7] Before dinner, you ought to walk on an empty stomach that retains no undigested food from earlier meals. You can tell if this is the case

ἐρευγμῶν ἀνοσμίᾳ καὶ ἐκλείψει καὶ τῇ λαπαρότητι καὶ τῇ εὐκρινείᾳ τοῦ ὑποχονδρίου καὶ τῆς κοιλίας, ἔτι δὲ τῷ πρὸς τὴν τοῦ φαγεῖν βούλησιν ὁρμητικῶς ἔχειν. δειπνεῖν δὲ καλῶς ἔχει τοῦ θέρους μικρὸν πρὸ ἡλίου δυσμῶν καὶ ἄρτον καὶ λάχανα καὶ μᾶζαν. λάχανα δ᾽ ὠμὰ μὲν προεσθίειν πλὴν σικύου καὶ ῥαφάνου (ταῦτα δὲ τελευταῖα), τὰ δ᾽ ἑφθὰ λαμβάνειν ὑπὸ πρῶτον τὸ δεῖπνον. ἰχθῦς δ᾽ ἐσθίειν τῶν μὲν πετραίων τοὺς σαρκώδεις καὶ ψαθυρούς, τῶν δὲ σελάχων καὶ τῶν ἄλλων τοὺς εὐχυλοτάτους καὶ πλεῖον τοὺς ἑφθούς· κρέα δ᾽ ἐρίφεια καὶ ἄρνεια τῶν νέων πάνυ, ὕεια δὲ τῶν ἀκμαζόντων, ὀρνίθεια δὲ τὰ τῶν ἀλεκτορίδων ἢ περδίκων ἢ περιστερῶν ἢ φαττῶν νεοττῶν, ἑφθὰ πάντα λιτῶς. λαμβάνειν δὲ καὶ τῶν ἄλλων ἐδεσμάτων οὐθὲν ἂν κωλύοι τὰ πρὸς ἡδονήν, ὅσα μὴ τοῖς προειρημένοις ἐναντίας ἔλαχε δυνάμεις. ὅτι δ᾽ ἁρμόττει πᾶσαν ὥραν τοῖς μὲν ὑγρὰς ἔχουσι τὰς κοιλίας <τὰ> στατικὰ λαμβάνειν τῶν παρόντων, τοῖς δὲ ξηρὰς τὰ ὑπακτικά, τοῖς δὲ δυσουροῦσι τὰ οὑρητικά, τοῖς δ᾽ ἰσχνοῖς τὰ τρόφιμα, πᾶς τις ἂν διδοίη. προπίνειν δὲ πρὸ τοῦ

most accurately from a lack of smell in your belches or a lack of belching altogether and from a looseness and lightness around the diaphragm and the bowels; another indication is having an appetite and desire for food. It is beneficial to eat a little bit before sunset in the summer: dine on bread and vegetables and barley cakes. Raw vegetables should be eaten as an appetizer to the meal (except for cucumber and kale—these should come at the end), whereas you should take boiled ones as part of the first course. When it comes to fish, eat rockfish that are fleshy and flaky, whereas cartilaginous ones and other kinds should be extremely succulent and usually stewed. As for meat, kid or lamb should be very young, pork should be from a pig in the prime of life, poultry should be a young chicken, partridge, pigeon, or ringdove, all simply boiled. As for other foods, nothing should stop you from taking what will give you pleasure, provided it doesn't have characteristics opposite to the ones just described. Anyone would tell you that, no

δείπνου καὶ πίνειν μέχρι τινὸς ὕδωρ· ἔπειτα τοὺς
μὲν ἰσχνοὺς [προπίνειν δὲ πρὸ τοῦ δείπνου] μέλανα λεπτὸν οἶνον, μετὰ δὲ τὸ δεῖπνον λευκόν,
τοὺς δ' εὐσάρκους διὰ τέλους λευκόν, ὑδαρέστερον δὲ πάντας, πλῆθος δ' ὅσον ἑκάστῳ γίνεται
πρὸς ἡδονήν. ἀκρόδρυα δὲ δύσχρηστα μέν ἐστι
πάντα, ἥκιστα δ' ἐνοχλεῖ τοῦ λόγου μέτρια λαμ-
βανόμενα πρὸ τῶν σιτίων. τῆς δ' ὀπώρας τὰ μὲν
σῦκα περιελόντας τὸ δέρμα καὶ τὸν ὀπὸν περι-
πλύναντας καὶ βρέξαντας ἐν ὕδατι ψυχρῷ βέλτιόν ἐστι λαμβάνειν, καὶ μὴ ἔχοντας αὐτοῦ καὶ
τοὺς μὴ δυναμένους ἐσθίειν μετὰ δεῖπνον, τοὺς
δὲ λοιποὺς πρὸ τοῦ δείπνου· σταφυλὴν δὲ λευ-
κὴν πάντας ἐν τῷ δείπνῳ· τραγήματα δ' ἐρεβίν-
θους λευκοὺς βεβρεγμένους ἢ ἀμύγδαλα καθαρὰ
βεβρεγμένα.

matter the season, it is suitable for those who have moist bowels to partake of whatever binding foods are available and for those with dry ones to eat ones that pass through easily; similarly, for those who have difficulty urinating to eat diuretic foods and for those who are thin to eat nourishing ones. Drink water before your meal and even a little bit into the beginning of it. Then, thin people should have a gentle, dark wine and, after the meal, a white one, whereas the well-fleshed should stick to white throughout, and all of it should be fairly watered-down; as for quantity, everyone should drink as much as gives them pleasure. Fruits from fruit trees are universally difficult; they cause the least trouble if you take a modest amount before your meal. In late summer, it is better to eat figs if you have first removed their skin, cleaned out their juice, and drenched them in cold water; anyone who doesn't have cold water and can't proceed accordingly should eat them after the meal; everyone else should eat them

[8] μετὰ δὲ τὸ δεῖπνον τοὺς μὲν ἰσχνοὺς καὶ φυσώδεις καὶ μὴ ῥᾳδίως τὰ σιτία πέττοντας ἁπλᾶ τε
λαμβάνειν καὶ καθεύδειν εὐθύς, τοὺς δὲ λοιποὺς
ὀλίγον καὶ βραδέως περιπατήσαντας ἀναπαύε-
σθαι. κεκλίσθαι δὲ παντὶ βέλτιόν ἐστι, ὄντος μὲν
ἔτι περὶ τὴν γαστέρα τοῦ πληρώματος, ἐπὶ τὴν
ἀριστερὰν πλευράν, λαπαρᾶς δὲ γενομένης μεταβάλλειν καὶ ἐπὶ τὴν δεξιάν· κατακεκλίσθαι δὲ
μήτε τεταμένον λίαν μήτε συγκεκαμμένον ἰσχυρῶς. ὕπτιον δὲ καθεύδειν οὐδενὶ βέλτιόν ἐστιν·
δύσπνοια γὰρ καὶ πνιγμοὶ καὶ ἐπιληπτικὰ καὶ ἐξ-
ονειριασμοὶ μάλιστα συμβαίνουσι τοῖς οὕτω κα-
θεύδουσιν. ἐγρηγορεῖν δὲ κατακειμένοις ὑπτίοις
τὸ μὲν γίνεται κατὰ τρόπον, τὸ δ' οὔ· τὰ μὲν γὰρ
σκέλη καὶ αἱ χεῖρες κατ' εὐθυωρίαν κείμενα τοῦ
σώματος πρὸς τὸ συγκάμπτειν καὶ ἐκτείνειν καὶ
συνάγειν καὶ διοίγειν εὖ ἔχει καὶ πρὸς τὸ τὰ δεξιὰ
τοῖς ἀριστεροῖς ὁμοίως κεῖσθαι, καὶ μὴ τὰ ἕτερα

before the meal. Everyone can eat a bunch of green grapes with dinner. As for after-dinner snacks, go for soaked white chickpeas or soaked blanched almonds.[3]

[8] After dinner, those who are thin or flatulent or who don't digest their food easily should take it easy and go to sleep immediately; everyone else can walk around gently for a little while before they rest. It is better in all cases to lie down on your left side while the bulk of the food is still in the region of your stomach; but once it empties out, to shift positions and lie on the right; don't stretch out too much when you lie down, but also don't be all tightly curled up. It is not advantageous for anyone to sleep on their back, since people who sleep in this way suffer especially from difficulty breathing, choking, epileptic fits, and nocturnal ejaculations. Lying on your back while still awake has both suitable and unsuitable aspects: the legs and the hands, lying in a straight line along the body instead of being doubled up, are well situated

θλίβεσθαι ὑπὸ τῶν ἑτέρων· ἡ δὲ ῥάχις πονεῖ διὰ τέλους ἐκτεταμένη παρὰ τὸ μὴ δυνατὸν εἶναι συγκάμπτειν αὐτὴν κατακειμένοις οὕτως. τὸ δ᾽ ὑποχόνδριον καὶ τοὺς πόδας ἀλεαίνειν οὐχ ἥκιστα ἁρμόττει παρά τε τὰ σιτία καὶ καθευδόντων. ἐγείρεσθαι μὲν καὶ ἀνίστασθαι τοὺς μὲν φυσώδεις ὀψέ, τοὺς δ᾽ ἄλλους ἅμα τῇ ἡμέρᾳ.*

[9] τοῖς μὲν οὖν πλείστοις τῶν ὑγιαινόντων τοιαύτη τις διαγωγὴ μάλιστα ἂν ἁρμόσειεν· τοῦ δὲ χειμῶνος ὅτι πλείω τοῦ θέρους τοὺς περιπάτους καὶ τὰ λοιπὰ γυμνάσια συντονώτερα δεῖ ποιεῖσθαι, κατὰ μικρὸν προσάγοντας, τὸ ἐπὶ πλεῖον εὐλαβουμένους, εἴρηται πρότερον. ἀλείμμασι δὲ

* van der Eijk's edition has this final sentence as the first sentence of section [9], but I felt it flowed better here, as the last sentence of section [8].

for bending down and stretching up and for coming together and opening out, and also easily allow for the right side to lie in the same way as the left instead of the one side being squashed by the other. On the other hand, the spine suffers from being completely stretched out in people who lie like this, because of not being able to bend itself. As for the abdomen and the feet, it is a matter of no small importance for them to be kept warm after food and while sleeping. The flatulent should wake up and rise on the late side; everyone else should get up at dawn.

[9] For most healthy people the following regimen for the winter would be the most suitable: walking should be more frequent than in summer and other gymnastic exercise should be done more strenuously, but ramp it up slowly and be cautious of overdoing it, as has been mentioned before. Use lotions more frequently than baths; use cold baths sometimes, especially on warm days, but, if you are fatigued and

μᾶλλον χρῆσθαι ἢ λουτροῖς· λουτροῖς δ᾽ ἐνίοτε
ψυχροῖς, καὶ μᾶλλον ἐν ταῖς θερμημερίαις,
θερμῷ δὲ τοὺς κοπιῶντας καὶ τοὺς ἀφιδρώσεως
δεομένους. καὶ τοὺς μὲν εὐσάρκους καὶ ὑγροὺς
ἁρμόττει [τε] μονοσιτεῖν ἀρξαμένους ἀπὸ Πλειά-
δος δύσεως <ἕως> ἐπιτολῆς· τοὺς δὲ λοιποὺς
ἀριστᾶν ἁρμόττει μικρὸν ὄψον ἔδοντας ἢ μέλι
μέτριον ἢ οἶνον γλυκύν, πίνειν δὲ μηδὲν ἢ μικρὸν
μετὰ τὸ ἄριστον οἰνάριον λεπτὸν ἀτρέμα μαλακόν, κεκιρναμένον μετρίως, ἔπειτα καταδαρθεῖν
ἀλεαίνοντας, μὴ πολὺν δὲ χρόνον· ἐγερθέντα δέ,
καθάπερ τοῦ θέρους, τὰ οἰκεῖα πράττειν, τὸ δὲ
λουτρὸν τὸ θερμὸν ἐᾶν, γυμνασαμένους δὲ δειπνεῖν συσκοτάζοντος, ἀλεαίνοντας μετὰ πυρός,
τοὺς μὲν μικροὺς καὶ εὖ πρὸς μᾶζαν ἔχοντας ἀμφότερα, πλείω δὲ τὸν ἄρτον, τοὺς δὲ λοιποὺς
ἀφαιρεῖν τὴν μᾶζαν. λάχανα δὲ τὸ μὲν ὅλον τοῦ
χειμῶνος <ἧττον> ἢ τοῦ θέρους ἐσθίειν ἁρμόττει.
μάλιστα δ᾽ εὐθετεῖ τῶν ὠμῶν οἷον πήγανον, εὔζωμον, ῥάφανος τελευταία λαμβανομένη· τῶν δ᾽
ἐφθῶν κράμβη, λάπαθον, γογγύλη, καὶ μᾶλλον
ἕωλος. τὰ δ᾽ ἄγρια, καὶ τὰ ὠμὰ τῶν ὠμῶν, καὶ τὰ

sweaty, you need a hot one. Fleshy and moist people ought to eat only one big meal a day in the period between the setting and the rising of the Pleiades constellation (that is, from early November to May). Everyone else ought to also eat a small lunch, with some relish or a modest amount of honey or sweet wine; drink nothing after the meal, or else have just a little bit of light, moderately mild wine, modestly diluted; then take a nap in a warm spot, but not for too long. When you wake up, go about your household business, just like in the summer, but skip the warm bath. Then, having exercised, eat dinner as it grows dark, warming yourself by the fire. Small people who enjoy barley cakes can eat both them and wheaten bread (more bread than cakes though); everyone else can skip the barley cakes. On the whole, it is a good idea to eat vegetables less frequently in the winter than in the summer. The most suitable raw vegetables are rue, arugula, and kale (if you eat it last in the meal); as for cooked ones: cabbage,[4]

ἑφθὰ τῶν ἑφθῶν, οὐ χείρω τὰ χειμερινὰ τῶν θε-
ρινῶν ἐστιν. ἁρμόττει δὲ καὶ τὰ σκόροδα καὶ τὰ
κρόμμυα καὶ ὁ τάριχος καὶ τὰ ἔτνη καὶ ἡ φακῆ μάλιστα ταύτην τὴν ὥραν, καὶ τῶν ἄλλων ὄψων μάλιστα τὰ ὀπτὰ τῶν ἑφθῶν, καὶ ὅλως τὰ ξηρότερα
τῶν ὑγροτέρων· χειμερινὸν δὲ <καὶ> τὸ κάρδαμον
καὶ τὸ σίνηπι μᾶλλόν ἐστιν. πίνειν δ᾽ ἐν μὲν τῷ δεί-
πνῳ οἶνον μέλανα, λεπτόν, ἡσυχῇ μαλακόν, μὴ
νέον, κιρνάμενον μικρὸν ἀκρατέστερον. ἁρμόττει
δὲ ταύτην τὴν ὥραν ἀμύγδαλα πεφρυγμένα,
μύρτα, βάλανοι ὀπτοί, κάρυα πλατέα, καὶ ἑφθὰ
καὶ ὀπτά.

[10] ὃν μὲν οὖν τρόπον δεῖ ζῆν τοῦ θέρους καὶ
τοῦ χειμῶνος, ἐπὶ πλεῖον εἴρηται· τοῦ δ᾽ ἔαρος καὶ
τοῦ φθινοπώρου δῆλον ὡς μέση δίαιτα τῶν εἰρημένων μάλιστα ἁρμόττει. φυλάττεσθαι δ᾽ ἀεὶ δεῖ
τά τε ἀήθη καὶ τὰ ἰσχυρὰ καὶ δύσπεπτα τῶν βρω-
μάτων καὶ τὰ πολλὰ λίαν· παρὰ γὰρ τὸ πλῆθος
οὐχ ἧττον ἢ παρὰ τὰς μοχθηρίας ἐνίοτε τῶν

patience dock,[5] and turnip (especially day-old). As for foraged ones, the winter plants are no worse than the summer ones (comparing the raw to the raw and the cooked to the cooked). The best foods in this season are garlic, onions, pickled fish, and thick bean or lentil soup; for the rest of your dishes, favor the roasted over the stewed and, in general, drier foods over moister ones. Pepperwort[6] and mustard are particularly wintery. During your meals, drink a red wine that is light, moderately gentle, not young, and mixed so that it's fairly undiluted. Desserts well-suited to the season are toasted almonds, myrtle berries, roasted acorns, and flat chestnuts (both boiled and roasted).

[10] Well then, the way you should live in both the summer and the winter has now been pretty much explained. As for spring and autumn, it should be obvious that you should follow a lifestyle halfway between the ones described. You must always be cautious about foods that are new to you or strong or difficult

ἐσθιομένων ἐνοχληθείη μᾶλλον ἄν τις. μὴ προ-
χείρως δὲ πίνειν ἄηθες ὕδωρ (μοχθηρὸν γὰρ καὶ
ἐπισφαλές ἐστιν), ἀλλὰ μετὰ μέλιτος ἢ οἴνου ἢ
ὄξους ἢ ἀλφίτων καὶ ἁλῶν. ψυχρὸν δ᾽ ἰσχυρῶς
ὕδωρ καὶ πάμπολυ πόμα ἀθροῦν πίνειν κινδυνῶ-
δές ἐστι, καὶ μάλιστα τοῖς πεπονηκόσι καὶ ἡλιου-
μένοις ἔτι θερμοῖς οὖσι. μέγιστον δὲ πρὸς ὑγίειάν
ἐστι τὸ μηδὲν κρεῖττον γίνεσθαι τῆς τοῦ σώματος φύσεως, ἅμα δὲ ταῖς ὥραις μεταβαλλούσαις
καὶ τὴν ἄλλην διαγωγὴν μεταβάλλειν, κατὰ μικρὸν εἰς τοὐναντίον ἀπονεύοντα, καὶ μὴ μεγά-
λην ἐξαπίνης ποιοῦντα μεταβολήν.

[11] ἀφροδισίοις δὲ χρῆσθαι πολλοῖς μὲν καὶ
συνεχὲς οὐ δεῖ· μάλιστα δ᾽ ἁρμόττει τοῖς ψυχροῖς
καὶ ὑγροῖς καὶ μελαγχολικοῖς καὶ φυσώδεσιν·
ἥκιστα δὲ κατὰ φύσιν μέν ἐστι τοῖς ἰσχνοῖς καὶ

to digest and about overindulging in most foods. In fact, people are no less likely to be troubled by the quantity of the food they eat than by its sometimes being of poor quality. Do not hastily drink water whose quality you are unfamiliar with (this is a pernicious and risky practice), but mix it with honey or wine or vinegar or barley meal and salt. It is dangerous to drink water (or really any beverage) that is extremely cold, especially so for people who have been exerting themselves or are still warm from being out in the sun. The best thing you can do for your health is to make sure that nothing that interacts with your body has a nature stronger than it, and, when the seasons change, change your lifestyle accordingly, being sure to gradually shift from one extreme to the other and never make a big change all of a sudden.

[11] As for sex, it is not a good idea to engage in too much all at once. It is most beneficial for cold, moist, melancholic, and flatulent people; least suitable for feeble or narrow-chested

ἀπλεύροις καὶ ἄσαρκα τὰ περὶ τὰ ἰσχία καὶ τὴν ὀσφὺν ἔχουσι, κατὰ δὲ τὰς ἡλικίας τοῖς ἐκ παίδων εἰς τὴν τῶν μειρακίων ἡλικίαν μεταβαίνουσι καὶ τοῖς πρεσβύταις. κακοῦται δὲ μάλιστα τοῦ σώματος τοῖς πλεονάζουσιν ἀκαίρως τὰ περὶ τὴν κύστιν καὶ νεφροὺς καὶ πνεύμονα καὶ ὀφθαλμοὺς καὶ τὰ περὶ τὸν νωτιαῖον μυελόν· ἥκιστα δ᾿ ἐνοχλεῖ καὶ πλεῖστον χρόνον ἡ δύναμις πρὸς ταῦτα διαμένει τοῖς μὴ ἄλλως ἀφυέσι πρὸς τὴν τοιαύτην πρᾶξιν ἐνεργοῦσί τε ἀεὶ μετρίως καὶ μὴ λίαν πλεονάζουσι, τροφῇ δὲ χρηστῇ καὶ δαψιλεῖ χρωμένοις.

people, for those who don't have much flesh around their hips and loins, and for those who are transitioning from childhood to adolescence, as well as for the elderly. The parts of the body most damaged by untimely overindulgence are the regions around the bladder, kidneys, lungs, and eyes, as well as those around the spinal marrow. Sex is least troublesome—and sexual endurance is most sustained—for those who are not otherwise unsuited to this sort of activity and who always engage in it moderately and not overfrequently, being sure to avail themselves of abundant, healthful food.

Celsus, *On Medicine* I.1–3

[1] Sanus homo, qui et bene valet et suae spontis est, nullis obligare se legibus debet, ac neque medico neque iatroalipta egere. Hunc oportet varium habere vitae genus: modo ruri esse, modo

SELF-CARE WITH CELSUS

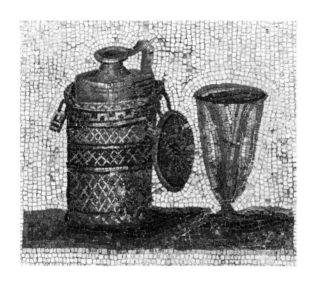

[1] A healthy person, who is both in good shape and a free agent, should have no need to live by special rules, nor require a doctor or a masseuse. Rather, he should lead a varied sort of life:

in urbe, saepiusque in agro; navigare, venari, quiescere interdum, sed frequentius se exercere; siquidem ignavia corpus hebetat, labor firmat, illa maturam senectutem, hic longam adulescentiam reddit.

Prodest etiam interdum balineo, interdum aquis frigidis uti; modo ungui, modo id ipsum neglegere; nullum genus cibi fugere, quo populus utatur; interdum in convictu esse, interdum ab eo se retrahere; modo plus iusto, modo non amplius adsumere; bis die potius quam semel cibum capere, et semper quam plurimum, dummodo hunc concoquat. Sed ut huius generis exercitationes cibique necessariae sunt, si<c> athletici supervacui: nam et intermissus propter civiles aliquas necessitates ordo exercitationis corpus adfligit, et ea corpora, quae more eorum repleta sunt, celerrime et senescunt et aegrotant. Concubitus vero neque nimis concupiscendus, neque nimis pertimescendus est. Rarus corpus

sometimes in the country, sometimes in the city, most often at home on his estate; he should sail and hunt and sometimes relax, but more often keep himself busy. Where laziness weakens the body, exertion firms it up: laziness makes you an old man before your time, but exertion keeps you teen-fit for years.

Some advice for this sort of person: sometimes take hot baths, sometimes cold; sometimes moisturize, sometimes skip it; don't avoid any type of normal food; sometimes be social, but sometimes withdraw for some alone time; sometimes take more than your share, but sometimes not so much; eat twice a day rather than just once, and always eat as much as you can manage and still digest it. Exercise and food of a normal sort are necessities, but athletes go over the top on both: if their exercise routine is interrupted even by some basic demand of society, the body suffers, and these same bodies quickly grow old and sick from their manner of gorging themselves. Sex shouldn't be too much

excitat, frequens solvit. Cum autem frequens non numero sit sed natura <aestimandus, habita> ratione aetatis et corporis, scire licet eum non inutilem esse, quem corporis neque languor neque dolor sequitur. Idem interdiu peior est, noctu tutior, ita tamen, si neque illum cibus, neque hunc cum vigilia labor statim sequitur. Haec firmis servanda sunt, cavendumque ne in secunda valetudine adversae praesidia consumantur.

[2] At inbecillis, quo in numero magna pars urbanorum omnesque paene cupidi litterarum sunt, observatio maior necessaria est, ut, quod vel corporis vel loci vel studii ratio detrahit, cura restituat. Ex his igitur qui bene concoxit, mane tuto surget; qui parum, quiescere debet, et si

of a focus, but also don't be too reticent about it. Done intermittently, it has a rousing effect on the body; done frequently, it loosens you up. But the frequency of sex should not be dictated by some number, but rather by your nature, depending on your age and temperament: a good rule of thumb is that you've got it right when sex leaves your body neither tired nor achy. Sex during the day is worse for you; sex at night is healthier; if you do it during the day, don't follow it with a meal; if you do it at night, don't stay awake and exert yourself right after. These are my tips to be followed by the healthy; and be careful that you don't squander your constitution's ability to resist adversity while you're in good health.

[2] For less robust people, however—and that includes the greater part of people who live in a city and almost everyone with academic inclinations—greater attention is required to ensure that they carefully counteract whatever in their bodies or location or studious lifestyle

mane surgendi necessitas fuit, redormire; qui non concoxit, ex toto conquiescere ac neque labori se neque exercitationi neque negotiis credere. Qui crudum sine praecordiorum dolore ructat, is ex intervallo aquam frigidam bibere, et se nihilo minus continere.

Habitare vero aedificio lucido, perflatum aestivum, hibernum solem habente; cavere meridianum solem, matutinum et vespertinum frigus, itemque auras fluminum atque stagnorum; minimeque nubilo caelo soli aperienti <subinde> se committere, ne modo frigus, modo calor moveat; quae res maxime gravedines destillationesque concitat. Magis vero gravibus locis ista

proves detrimental. For the people in this group: whoever has digested well can safely get up early in the morning; those who have digested insufficiently should stay in bed—and if something requires them to get up early, they should go back to sleep later; those who have not digested at all should remain in every way at rest and commit themselves neither to exertion nor to exercise nor to business. Anyone who belches up their food without feeling heartburn should drink cold water a little after and be particularly conscious about exercising self-restraint.

Advice for these people: live in a house that is full of light, airy in the summer, sunny in the winter. Be careful of noonday heat and of chills in the morning and the evening, as well as of the fumes of rivers and marshes. Don't expose yourself to weather when the sun comes in and out in a cloudy sky, which can make you alternatingly hot and cold: this particularly leads to stuffy noses and colds. You need to be even

servanda sunt, in quibus etiam pestilentiam faciunt.

Scire autem licet integrum corpus esse, quo die mane urina alba, dein rufa est: illud concoquere, hoc concoxisse significat. Ubi experrectus est aliquis, paulum intermittere; deinde, nisi hiemps est, fovere os multa aqua frigida debet; longis diebus meridiari potius ante cibum; si minus, post eum. Per hiemem potissimum totis noctibus conquiescere; sin lucubrandum est, non post cibum id facere, sed post concoctionem. Quem interdiu vel domestica vel civilia officia tenuerunt, huic tempus aliquod servandum curationi corporis sui est. Prima autem eius curatio exercitatio est, quae semper antecedere cibum debet, in eo, qui minus laboravit et bene concoxit, amplior; in eo, qui fatigatus est et minus concoxit, remissior.

more careful about this in unwholesome places, where it can even lead to pestilence.

You can know that your body is in good shape if your urine is pale in the morning and tawny later on: the first means you are digesting, the second that you have finished digesting. When you wake up, you should wait a little bit and then bathe your face with lots of cold water (unless it is winter). When the days are long, it is preferable to have your nap before lunch; as they grow shorter, have it after. In the winter, it is extremely important to get a full night's sleep. But if you must work into the night, don't do it right after dinner but wait until you have had a chance to digest. Anyone who has a job that keeps them busy during the day, whether in the private or the public sector, must still set aside some time for the care of their body. The most important aspect of this care is exercise, which should always be done before food: if you've had a light day and have digested well, push

Commode vero exercent clara lectio, arma, pila, cursus, ambulatio, atque haec non utique plana commodior est, siquidem melius ascensus quoque et descensus cum quadam varietate corpus moveat, nisi tamen id perquam inbecillum est: melior autem est sub divo quam in porticu; melior, si caput patitur, in sole quam in umbra, <melior in umbra> quam paries aut viridia efficiunt, quam quae tecto subest; melior recta quam flexuosa. Exercitationis autem plerumque finis esse debet sudor aut certe lassitudo, quae citra fatigationem sit, idque ipsum modo minus, modo magis faciendum est. Ac ne his quidem athletarum exemplo vel certa esse lex vel inmodicus labor debet. Exercitationem recte sequitur modo unctio, vel in sole vel ad ignem; modo balineum, sed conclavi quam maxime et alto et lucido et spatioso. Ex his vero neutrum semper fieri oportet, sed saepius alterutrum pro

yourself more; if you're tired and haven't digested as well, go easier.

Some convenient exercises: reading aloud, fencing, playing ball, running, walking. As for walking, it is better for you to do it on terrain that is not completely level because going uphill and downhill offers some variety and moves the body in a better way (unless it is exceedingly frail); better to walk out in open places rather than under a colonnade; better to walk in sun than in shade (assuming your head can handle it); if it has to be shade, better that of a wall or of greenery than under a roof; better in a straight line than on a windy path. For the most part, you know you've come to the end of your exercise when you are sweaty or at least tired, but not so tired that you're exhausted: sometimes you need to do more, sometimes less. People in this category should absolutely not try to model themselves after athletes and do strict training programs or an immoderate amount of exertion.

corporis natura. Post haec paulum conquiescere opus est.

Ubi ad cibum ventum est, numquam utilis est nimia satietas, saepe inutilis nimia abstinentia: si qua intemperantia subest, tutior est in potione quam in esca. Cibus a salsamentis, holeribus similibusque rebus melius incipit; tum caro adsumenda est, quae assa optima aut elixa est. Condita omnia duabus causis inutilia sunt, quoniam et plus propter dulcedinem adsumitur, et quod modo par est, tamen aegrius concoquitur. Secunda mensa bono stomacho nihil nocet, in inbecillo coacescit. Si quis itaque hoc parum valet, palmulas pomaque et similia melius primo cibo adsumit. Post multas potiones, quae aliquantum

Exercise should properly be followed sometimes by moisturizing (either in the sun or in front of a fire), sometimes by a bath (but it should be in a really big bathroom: high ceilinged, bright, and spacious). You should certainly not stick to one of these options invariably, but you should favor whichever one is better suited to the nature of your body. After all this, you must rest for a bit.

When it comes to food, excessive abundance is never good, and excessive abstinence is often bad: if some intemperance is on the horizon, it is safer for it to be related to beverages than to food. A meal is best begun with pickled fish, vegetables, and similar things; then meat should be taken, which has ideally been either roasted or stewed. All culinary concoctions are bad for two reasons: both because more of them is eaten due to their palatability and because even an appropriate amount of them is still digested in an unhealthy way. The dessert course does no harm to a strong stomach, but it turns sour in a weak

sitim excesserunt, nihil edendum est, post satietatem nihil agendum. Ubi expletus est aliquis, facilius concoquit, si, quicquid adsumpsit, potione aquae frigidae includit, tum paulisper invigilat, deinde bene dormit. Si quis interdiu se inplevit, post cibum neque frigori neque aestui neque labori se debet committere: neque enim tam facile haec inani corpore quam repleto nocent. Si quibus de causis futura inedia est, labor omnis vitandus est.

[3] Atque haec quidem paene perpetua sunt. Quasdam autem observationes desiderant <et> novae res et corporum genera et sexus et aetates et tempora anni. . . . Neque ex multa vero fame nimia satietas neque ex nimia satietate fames idonea est. Periclitaturque et qui semel et qui bis die cibum incontinenter contra consuetudinem

one: anyone who is insufficiently hearty in this regard would do better to take his dates, apples, and the like before dinner. After overindulgence in drinks (more than thirst demanded), no food should be consumed; after abundant food, stay idle. When a person is stuffed, he more easily digests if he includes a drink of cold water with whatever he has eaten, stays awake for a bit afterward, and then sleeps soundly. If someone stuffs himself at lunchtime, he ought to expose himself neither to the cold nor to the heat nor to exertion: for these do not as easily harm an empty body as they do a full one. If for whatever reason you foresee a period of fasting, every exertion must be avoided.

[3] The advice above should just about last you a lifetime. However, a few further observations are worthwhile with regard to transitions, as well as to body types, gender, age, and season of the year. . . . It is not a good idea to be too indulgent after extended fasting, nor to fast after overindulgence. It is risky to take two big

adsumit. Item neque ex nimio labore subitum otium neque ex nimio otio subitus labor sine gravi noxa est. Ergo cum quis mutare aliquid volet, paulatim debebit adsuescere.

Omnem etiam laborem facilius vel puer vel senex quam insuetus homo sustinet. Atque ideo quoque nimis otiosa vita utilis non est, quia potest incidere laboris necessitas. Si quando tamen insuetus aliquis laboravit, aut si multo plus quam solet etiam si qui adsuevit, huic ieiuno dormiendum est, multo magis etiam si os amarum est vel oculi caligant, aut venter perturbatur: tum enim non dormiendum tantummodo ieiuno est, sed etiam <quieto> in posterum diem permanendum, nisi cito id quies sustulit. Quod si factum est, surgere oportet et lente paulum ambulare. At si somni necessitas non fuit, quia modice magis aliquis laboravit, tamen ingredi aliquid eodem modo debet.

meals a day when you're used to one, or one when you're used to two. Similarly, you can't go from overexertion to sudden rest, nor from extended rest straight to exertion without serious bad effects. In short, whenever you want to change something, accustom yourself to it gradually.

Even a child or an old man can do a job more easily than a man who is not used to exertion. For that reason, it is not a good idea to lead too idle a life because you never know when you might be forced to exert yourself. That said, if you ever have to exert yourself contrary to custom—or more than you are accustomed to do—you should go to sleep on an empty stomach. All the more so if you have a bitter taste in your mouth or your vision goes dark or your stomach is upset—in that case, don't just go to bed on an empty stomach, but also spend the next day taking it easy; unless rest immediately improved things, in which case it's okay to get up and slowly take a little stroll. Even if sleep

Communia deinde omnibus sunt post fatigationem cibum sumpturis: ubi paulum ambu-
laverunt, si balneum non est, calido loco vel in sole
vel ad ignem ungui atque sudare; si est, ante
omnia in tepidario sedere, deinde ubi paululum
conquierunt, intrare et descendere in solium;
tum multo oleo ungui leniterque perfricari,
iterum in solium descendere, post haec os aqua
calida, deinde frigida fovere. Balineum his fervens
idoneum non est. . . . Post haec omnibus fatigatis
aptum est cibum sumere, eoque umido uti, aqua
vel certe diluta potione esse contentos, maximeque
ea, quae moveat urinam. Illud quoque nosse
oportet, quod ex labore sudanti frigida potio
perniciosissima est . . .

was not necessary, because you only exerted yourself slightly more than normal, you should still take a little stroll like this.

In fact, here's a general rule for anyone who is going to eat after doing something tiring: first take a little walk; then, if there is no bathhouse handy, go to some hot place—in the sun, or near the fire—put on some lotion and sweat; if there is a bathhouse, start out first thing by sitting in the warm room, then once you've rested there for a little bit, go take a dip in the tub. Then get gently rubbed down with a lot of oil and get back in the tub again. Afterward, wash your face, first in hot water, then in cold. A very hot bath is not appropriate in this sort of situation. . . . After doing these things, it is okay for fatigued people to eat some food, but they should stick to a liquid diet and be content with drinking either water or a diluted drink (one that really gets the urine going would be great). It is also wise to know that a cold drink

Si adsidua fatigatio urguet, in vicem modo aquam, modo vinum bibendum est, raro balineo utendum. Levatque lassitudinem etiam laboris mutatio; eumque, quem novum genus eiusdem laboris pressit, id quod in consuetudine est, reficit. Fatigato cotidianum cubile tutissimum est: lassat enim quod contra consuetudinem, seu molle seu durum est. . . . Qui vero toto die vel in vehiculo vel in spectaculis sedit, huic nihil currendum sed lente ambulandum est. Lenta quoque in balineo mora, dein cena exigua prodesse consuerunt. . . .

Ante omnia autem norit quisque naturam sui corporis, quoniam alii graciles, alii obessi sunt, alii calidi, alii frigidiores, alii umidi, alii sicci; alios adstricta, alios resoluta alvus exercet. Raro quisquam non aliquam partem corporis inbecil-

is the worst thing you can take after sweating from exertion. . . .

If you are afflicted by constant fatigue, you should alternate drinking wine and water and use the bathhouse only rarely. A change in exertion can actually lighten weariness: if some new type of exertion is tiring you, going back to your accustomed one can refresh you. For a tired person, the bed you're used to sleeping in is the safest one for you: an unfamiliar mattress will weary you, no matter whether it is soft or hard. . . . For anyone who spent the whole day sitting, either in a carriage or at a show: definitely do not go for a run; have a gentle walk instead. It is a good idea to while away some time in the bathhouse, and then have a light dinner. . . .

The most important thing of all, though, is that everyone should be familiar with the nature of their own body: some people are underweight, others are over; some naturally run hot, others cold; some are naturally moist,

lam habet. Tenuis vero homo inplere se debet, plenus extenuare; calidus refrigerare, frigidus calefacere; madens siccare, siccus madefacere; itemque alvum firmare is, cui fusa, solvere is, cui adstricta est: succurrendumque semper parti maxime laboranti est.

Implet autem corpus modica exercitatio, frequentior quies, unctio et, si post prandium est, balineum; contracta alvus, modicum frigus hieme, somnus et plenus et non nimis longus, molle cubile, animi securitas, adsumpta per cibos et potiones maxime dulcia et pinguia; cibus et frequentior et quantus plenissimus potest concoqui. Extenuat corpus aqua calida, si quis in ea descendit, magisque si salsa est; ieiuno

others dry; some people's bowels incline to be constipated, others' run too freely. It is rare for anyone to not have some part of his body that is a weak point. The thin person needs to bulk himself up, the stout to thin himself down. The person who runs hot needs to cool himself down; the one who runs cold to warm himself up. The moist person needs to dry out, the dry to get moister. An incontinent person needs to tighten up their bowels, a constipated one to relax them. Basically, whichever part is most problematic should always get the most attention.

Things to bulk up the body: modest exercise, more frequent rest, moisturizing, and visits to the bathhouse (but only after lunch). Keep the bowels tight; don't get too cold in the winter; get plenty of sleep, but don't sleep for too long at a time; use a soft mattress. No stress. Pick food and drinks with the most sugar and fat content; eat more frequently and eat as much as you can and still digest it. Things to thin down

balineum, inurens sol ut omnis calor, cura, vigilia;
somnus nimium vel brevis vel longus, per aestatem
durum cubile; cursus, multa ambulatio, omnisque
vehemens exercitatio; vomitus, deiectio, acidae
res et austerae; et semel die adsumptae epulae; et
vini non praefrigidi ieiuno potio in consuetudinem
adducta. . . .

Calefacit autem unctio, aqua salsa, magisque
si calida est, omnia salsa, amara, carnosa; si post
cibum est, balneum, vinum austerum. Refrigerant
in ieiunio et balneum et somnus, nisi nimis longus
est, omnia acida, aqua <quam> frigidissima,
oleum, si aqua miscetur.

Umidum autem corpus efficit labor maior
quam ex consuetudine, frequens balineum, cibus
plenior, multa potio, post hanc ambulatio et
vigilia; per se quoque ambulatio multa et matutina
et vehemens, exercitationi non protinus cibus

the body: baths in hot water (especially saltwater), baths on an empty stomach; blazing sun (or really any heat); worry, staying up late; periods of sleep that run either too short or too long, a hard bed in the summer; running, lots of walking, and any kind of strenuous exercise; vomiting, enemas, eating sour and tart things. Eat one big meal a day and make a habit of drinking wine (not too cold) on an empty stomach. . . .

Things to warm the body: moisturizing, saltwater (especially if it's hot); all salty, bitter, and meaty food; baths (but only after food); tart wine. Things to cool the body: both bathing and sleeping while fasting (as long as the period of sleep is not too long); all acidic foods, water as cold as possible; moisturizing (but only with watered-down oil).

Things to moisten the body: more exertion than customary, frequent visits to the bathhouse; more abundant food and lots to drink, followed by walking and not sleeping. Also just walking on its own (do it a lot, early in the

adiectus; ea genera escae, quae veniunt ex locis frigidis et pluviis et inriguis. Contra siccat modica exercitatio, fames, unctio sine aqua, calor, sol modicus, frigida aqua, cibus exercitationi statim subiectus, et is ipse ex siccis et aestuosis locis veniens.

Alvum adstringit labor, sedile, creta figularis corpori inlita, cibus inminutus, et is ipse semel die adsumptus ab eo, qui bis solet; exigua potio neque adhibita, nisi cum cibi quis, quantum adsumpturus est, cepit, post cibum quies. Contra solvit aucta ambulatio atque esca po<tusque>, motus, qui post cibum est, subinde potiones cibo inmixtae. . . .

Quod ad aetates vero pertinet, inediam facillime sustinent mediae aetates, minus iuvenes, minime pueri et senectute confecti. Quo minus fert facile quisque, eo saepius debet cibum

morning, and vigorously). Don't immediately eat after exercise; foods should come from cold, rainy, well-irrigated places. In contrast, things to dry the body: modest exercise, hunger, moisturizing with undiluted oil, heat, moderate sunshine, cold water. Take food immediately after exercise, and it should come from dry, hot places.

Things to tighten the bowels: exertion, sitting in hard chairs, mud treatments; an undiminished amount of food (but eaten all in one big meal rather than in two, if that's what you were accustomed to), not much to drink (unless you drink everything you're going to drink with the meal), rest after food. In contrast, things to loosen the bowels: increased walking and food and drink, movement after meals, undiluted drinks immediately after food. . . .

As for the topic of age: middle-aged people tolerate fasting most easily, younger people less so, children and the elderly least of all. The less easily one tolerates fasting, the more frequently

adsumere, maximeque eo eget, qui increscit. Calida lavatio et pueris et senibus apta est. Vinum dilutius pueris, senibus meracius: neutri aetati, quae inflationes movent. Iuvenum minus quae adsumant et quomodo curentur, interest. Quibus iuvenibus fluxit alvus, plerumque in senectute contrahitur: quibus in adulescentia fuit adstricta, saepe in senectute solvitur. Melior est autem in iuvene fusior, in sene adstrictior.

Tempus quoque anni considerare oportet. Hieme plus esse convenit, minus sed meracius bibere; multo pane uti, carne potius elixa, modice holeribus; semel <die> cibum capere, nisi si nimis venter adstrictus est. Si prandet aliquis, utilius est exiguum aliquid, et ipsum siccum sine carne, sine potione sumere. Eo tempore anni calidis omnibus

one should eat; someone who is growing should eat most frequently of all. Warm baths are suitable to both children and the elderly. Children should have fairly diluted wine, the elderly fairly neat: neither group should have wine that causes gas. Young adults are more resilient as to what they eat and how. Anyone who has loose bowels in their youth will see them tighten up as they get elderly; whereas those who are constipated as teenagers often see things loosen up as they get elderly. But the better situation is to be on the looser side in youth and on the tighter side in old age.

It is also a good idea to consider the time of year. Tips for the winter: eat more and drink less (but less diluted); eat lots of bread, meat that's mostly stewed, and a modest amount of vegetables; eat one big meal a day (unless your stomach is too small). If you also eat a lunch, it is better to partake of something small and dry: no meat, no beverage. At this time of year, everything you consume should tend to be hot or

potius utendum est vel calorem moventibus.
Venus tum non aeque perniciosa est. At vere
paulum cibo demendum, adiciendum potioni,
sed dilutius tamen bibendum est; magis carne
utendum, magis holeribus; transeundum paulatim
ad assa ab elixis. Venus eo tempore anni tutissima
est. Aestate vero et potione et cibo saepius corpus
eget; ideo prandere quoque commodum est. Ei
tempori aptissima sunt et caro et holus, potio
quam dilutissima, ut et sitim tollat nec corpus
incendat; frigida lavatio, caro assa, frigidi cibi vel
qui refrigerent. Ut saepius autem cibo utendum,
sic exiguo est. Per autumnum propter caeli
varietatem periculum maximum est. Itaque neque
sine veste neque sine calciamentis prodire
oportet, praecipueque diebus frigidioribus, neque
sub divo nocte dormire, aut certe bene operiri.
Cibo vero iam paulo pleniore uti licet, minus sed
meracius bibere. . . . Neque aestate vero neque
autumno utilis venus est, tolerabilior tamen per

heat-producing. Sex at this time tends to not be as pernicious as it can be. But in the spring, diminish the amount of food you eat a bit and increase the amount that you drink (but the drinks should be pretty diluted); avail yourself of more meat and more vegetables; gradually shift from stewed foods to roasted ones. Sex is at its safest at this time of year. In the summer, the body requires both food and drink frequently; therefore, it is a good idea to eat a lunch. At this time of year, meat and vegetables are the best foods, and drink should be at its most diluted (so that it takes away thirst without overheating the body); baths should be cold, meat roasted, foods either cold or cooling. But because you are eating more frequently, you should accordingly eat small portions. Autumn is the most dangerous time of year because the weather is changeable. Therefore, you should never venture out without both a warm layer and shoes, especially on colder days, and don't sleep out in the open at night (or at least keep

autumnum: aestate in totum, si fieri potest, abstinendum est.

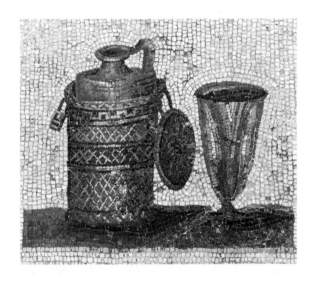

well covered if you do). It is now okay to take a little more food, and drink a little less (and less diluted). . . . Sex is not a good idea in summer or in autumn; it's more tolerable in the autumn, but you should abstain from it altogether in the summer, if you can stand to.

Part II

What to Eat

Radishes

ὠμὴν μὲν αὐτὴν ἐσθίουσι μόνην τοὐπίπαν
οἱ κατὰ τὰς πόλεις ἄνθρωποι πρώτην ἁπάντων μετὰ γάρου γαστρὸς ὑπαγωγῆς ἕνεκεν, ὀλίγοι δὲ καὶ ὄξους ἐπιχέουσιν. οἱ δ᾽
ἐν τοῖς ἀγροῖς καὶ μετ᾽ ἄρτου πολλάκις
προσφέρονται παραπλησίως τοῖς ἄλλοις
αὐτοφυέσιν ὄψοις, ἐξ ὧν ἐστι καὶ ὀρίγανος

APPETIZERS AND RELISHES

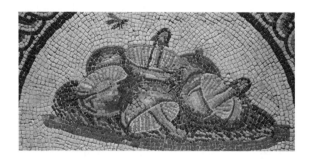

Radishes

City-folk usually eat these raw with some fish sauce on their own before a meal in order to clear out their stomachs; a few people also like them with vinegar. Country-folk often also serve them with bread, like they do with other locally grown relishes — for example, fresh oregano, pepperwort,

ἡ χλωρὰ καὶ κάρδαμον καὶ θύμα καὶ θύμβρα καὶ γλήχων καὶ ἕρπυλλος ἡδύοσμός τε καὶ καλαμίνθη καὶ πύρεθρον καὶ εὔζωμον. ἅπαντα γὰρ ταῦτα τῶν ἐδωδίμων ἐστὶν ὄψα χλωρὰ μετὰ τῶν τροφῶν ἐσθιόμενα, τῶν ποωδῶν φυτῶν ὄντα.

—Galen, *De alimentorum facultatibus* II.68 (VI.656–57K)

ὑπὸ ῥαφανίδος τρεφόμεθα μέν, ἀλλ᾽ οὐχ ὡς ὑπὸ τῶν κρεῶν. ... ἐν δὲ τῇ ῥαφανίδι τὸ μὲν οἰκεῖόν τε καὶ μεταβληθῆναι δυνάμενον, μόγις καὶ τοῦτο καὶ σὺν πολλῇ τῇ κατεργασίᾳ, παντάπασιν ἐλάχιστον· ὅλη δ᾽ ὀλίγου δεῖν ἐστι περιττωματικὴ καὶ διεξέρχεται τὰ τῆς πέψεως ὄργανα, βραχέος ἐξ αὐτῆς εἰς τὰς φλέβας ἀναληφθέντος αἵματος καὶ οὐδὲ τούτου τελέως χρηστοῦ.

—Galen, *De naturalibus facultatibus* I.10 (II.22K)

thyme, savory, pennyroyal, flowering thyme, mint and catmint, Spanish chamomile, and arugula. For all of these sorts of food, being herb-like plants, serve as fresh relishes to be eaten as a compliment to meals.

— Galen, *On the Properties of Foodstuffs*

We are nourished by the radish, but not to the same degree that we are by meat. . . . In the radish, the part that is compatible with us and able to be altered — and barely, at that, and with a great deal of work — is quite minuscule; almost all of the radish results in residues and passes through and out the organs of digestion, with only a small part of it being taken up into the veins as blood, and this blood is not fully useable.

— Galen, *On the Natural Faculties*

ῥαφανὶς καὶ αὐτὴ πνευμάτων γεννητική, εὔστομος, οὐκ εὐστόμαχος, ἐρευκτική. οὐρητικὴ δὲ ἐστι καὶ θερμαντική, εὐκοίλιος δέ, εἴ τις αὐτὴν ἐπιλαμβάνει μᾶλλον συν-εργοῦσαν τῇ ἀναδόσει, προεσθιομένη δὲ μετεωρίζει τὴν τροφήν.

—Dioscorides, *De materia medica* II.112

Amaritudo plurima illis est et pro crassitudine corticis. Cetera quoque aliquando lignosa. Et vis mira colligendi spiritum laxandique ructum; ob id cibus inliberalis . . . Utilissimi in cibis hiberno tempore existimantur, iidemque dentibus semper inimici, quoniam adterant: ebora certe poliunt.

—Pliny the Elder, *Naturalis historia* XIX.26.78–79, 87

The radish is productive of flatulence; it is easy on the tastebuds but not on the stomach; it causes burping. It is also diuretic and warming. It is good for the bowels if you have it after other food, when it is more helpful to digestion; but if you eat if before your meal, it makes your food come back up.

—Dioscorides, *Medical Substances*

There is a great deal of bitterness in these, proportional to the thickness of their skin. The rest of the radish is sometimes also woody. And they have a remarkable power to produce gas and let out belches; as a result, this is a lower-class food. . . . They are considered most useful as food in the winter, though they are always hard on the teeth: in fact, they make a good ivory polish.

—Pliny the Elder, *Natural History*

Olives

ὀλίγην μὲν πάνυ καὶ αὗται τροφὴν διδόασι
τῷ σώματι καὶ μάλισθ᾽ αἱ δρυπεπεῖς. ἐσθίουσι δ᾽ οἱ ἄνθρωποι ταύτας μὲν σὺν ἄρτῳ
μᾶλλον, ἄνευ δ᾽ ἄρτου τὰς ἁλμάδας τὲ καὶ
κολυμβάδας ὀνομαζομένας ἕνεκα γαστρὸς
ὑπαγωγῆς μετὰ γάρου πρὸ τῶν σιτίων.
ὥσπερ δ᾽ αἱ δρυπεπεῖς πλεῖστον τὸν λιπαρόν, οὕτως αὗται τὸν στύφοντα χυμὸν
ἔχουσι. διὸ καὶ ῥωννύουσι τὸν στόμαχον
ἐπεγείρουσί τε τὴν ὄρεξιν. ἐπιτηδειόταται δ᾽
εἰς τοῦτ᾽ εἰσὶν αἱ μετ᾽ ὄξους ἀποτιθέμεναι.

—Galen, *De alimentorum facultatibus* II.27
(VI.608–9K)

Capers

ταράττει δὲ κοιλίαν, κακοστόμαχός τε
ἐστι καὶ διψώδης, βρωθεῖσα δὲ ἐφθὴ
εὐστομαχωτέρα τῆς ὠμῆς. . . . ὀδόντος

Olives

These provide very little nourishment to the body, especially the tree-ripened ones. People usually eat them with bread; but they eat the ones known as "salted-and-swimming" without bread before their meals with some fish sauce in order to clear out their stomachs. While the tree-ripened ones are the oiliest, these have a binding juice. As a result, they strengthen the stomach and stimulate the appetite. The ones pickled in vinegar are best suited to do this.

—Galen, *On the Properties of Foodstuffs*

Capers

The caper troubles the bowels, is bad for the stomach, and makes you thirsty. It is easier on the stomach if eaten boiled than

πόνον παύει ὁ καρπὸς σὺν ὄξει ἑψηθεὶς
καὶ διακλυζόμενος.

—Dioscorides, *De materia medica* II.173

χρώμεθα δ᾽ ὡς φαρμάκῳ μᾶλλον ἢ ὡς
τροφῇ τῷ καρπῷ τοῦ φυτοῦ. κομίζεται γὰρ
ὡς ἡμᾶς ἁλσὶ διαπασθεῖσα διὰ τὸ σήπε-
σθαι μόνην ἀποτιθεμένην. εὔδηλον οὖν ὅτι
χλωρὰ μὲν ἔτι πρὶν ταριχευθῆναι πλέον
ἔχει τροφῆς. ἐκ δὲ τῆς ταριχείας ἀπόλλυσι
πάμπολυ καὶ γίγνεται χωρὶς μὲν τοῦ τοὺς
ἅλας ἀποπλυθῆναι παντάπασιν ἄτροφος,
ὑπακτικὴ δὲ τῆς γαστρός· ἀποπλυθεῖσα δὲ
καὶ διαβραχεῖσα μέχρι τοῦ τελέως ἀποθέ-
σθαι τὴν ἐκ τῶν ἁλῶν δύναμιν, ὡς ἔδεσμα
μὲν ὀλιγοτροφώτατόν ἐστιν, ὡς ὄψον δὲ
καὶ φάρμακον ἐπιτήδειον ἐπεγεῖραι κατα-
πεπτωκυῖαν ὄρεξιν ἀπορρύψαι τε καὶ ὑπα-
γαγεῖν τὸ κατὰ τὴν γαστέρα φλέγμα καὶ

if eaten raw. ... The fruit stops tooth-
aches if you boil it with vinegar and use it
as a mouthwash.

—Dioscorides, *Medical Substances*

We use the fruit of this plant more as a
drug than a food. It is imported to us preserved in salt because it rots if packed
plain. Obviously, it is more nutritious
while still fresh, before being pickled. If
you take it right from its pickling juice
without washing away the salt, it is completely worthless as a food, though it does
clear out the stomach. But washed and
soaked until the potency of the salt has
completely gone away, it still offers only a
minuscule amount of nourishment as a
food but is useful as a relish and as a drug
to stimulate an appetite for food and to
cleanse and carry off phlegm from the

τὰς κατὰ σπλῆνα καὶ ἧπαρ ἐμφράξεις ἐκκαθῆραι.

—Galen, *De alimentorum facultatibus* II.34 (VI.615–16K)

Basil

ὄψῳ μὲν καὶ τούτῳ χρῶνται πολλοὶ δι' ἐλαίου καὶ γάρου προσφερόμενοι, κακοχυμότατον δ' ἐστὶ καὶ διὰ τοῦτο προσεπικαταψεύδονταί τινες αὐτοῦ φάσκοντες, εἰ τριφθὲν ἐμβληθείη χύτρᾳ καινῇ, τάχιστα γεννᾶν ἐν ὀλίγαις ἡμέραις σκορπίους, καὶ μάλισθ' ὅταν ἐν ἡλίῳ τις ἑκάστης ἡμέρας θερμαίνῃ τὴν χύτραν. ἀλλὰ τοῦτο μὲν ψεῦδός ἐστι, κακόχυμον δὲ καὶ κακοστόμαχον καὶ δύσπεπτον εἶναι λάχανον ἀληθῶς ἂν εἴποις αὐτό.

—Galen, *De alimentorum facultatibus* II.55 (VI.640–41K)

stomach and clear out stoppages in the spleen and liver.

—Galen, *On the Properties of Foodstuffs*

Basil

Many people serve this as a relish with olive oil and fish sauce, but it is extremely unwholesome, and for this reason some people make the ridiculous claim that, if you grind it up and put it in a newly made pot, scorpions will spring into being from it within a few days, especially if you leave the pot to warm in the sun every day. While that is false, it is certainly true to say that it is an unwholesome vegetable, bad for the stomach and for digestion.

—Galen, *On the Properties of Foodstuffs*

ὤκιμον βιβρωσκόμενον πολὺ ἀμβλυωπές
ἐστιν. ἔστι δὲ κοιλίας μαλακτικόν, πνευμάτων κινητικόν, οὐρητικόν, γάλακτος προ-
κλητικόν, δυσμετάβλητον. . . . φυλάσσονται
δέ τινες αὐτὸ καὶ οὐχ ἐσθίουσι διὰ τὸ μαση-
θὲν καὶ τεθὲν ἐν ἡλίῳ σκώληκας γεννᾶν.
Λίβυες δὲ προσυπειλήφασιν, ὅτι οἱ φαγόντες
αὐτὸ καὶ πληγέντες ὑπὸ σκορπίου ἀσώστως
διατίθενται.

—Dioscorides, *De materia medica* II.141

Mushrooms

Ostreis boletisque in omnem vitam re-
nuntiatum est; nec enim cibi sed oblecta-
menta sunt ad edendum saturos cogentia
(quod gratissimum est edacibus et se ultra
quam capiunt farcientibus), facile descen-
sura, facile reditura!

—Seneca, *Epistulae* 108.15

Basil eaten in too great a quantity causes dim-sightedness. It is softening to the bowels, productive of flatulence, diuretic, stimulating for milk-production, and difficult to digest. . . . Some people are wary of it and do not eat it because it grows worms if you mash it up and leave it in the sun. The Libyans further believe that those who eat it and then get struck by a scorpion are unable to be saved.

—Dioscorides, *Medical Substances*

Mushrooms

I have sworn off oysters and mushrooms forever. For they are not food, but relishes that compel full people to eat more (which is the ultimate pleasure for gluttons and those who stuff their faces with more than they can handle)—easy in, easy out!

—Seneca, *Letters*

καὶ τῶν μυκήτων οἱ βωλῖται, καλῶς ἑψηθέ-
ντες ἐν ὕδατι, πλησίον ἥκουσι τῶν ἀποίων
ἐδεσμάτων. οὐ μὴν οὕτω γε μόνοις αὐτοῖς
οἱ ἄνθρωποι χρῶνται, σκευάζουσι δὲ καὶ
ἀρτύουσι πολυειδῶς, ὥσπερ καὶ τἄλλα, ὅσα
μηδεμίαν ἐξαίρετον ἔχει ποιότητα. φλεγμα-
τώδης δ' ἐστὶν ἡ ἐξ αὐτῶν τροφὴ καὶ δῆλον
ὅτι καὶ ψυχρά, κἂν πλεονάζῃ τις ἐν αὐτοῖς,
κακόχυμος. ἀβλαβέστατοι μὲν οὖν τῶν
ἄλλων μυκήτων εἰσὶν οὗτοι, δεύτεροι δὲ μετ'
αὐτοὺς οἱ ἀμανῖται. τῶν δ' ἄλλων ἀσφαλέ-
στερόν ἐστι μηδ' ὅλως ἅπτεσθαι· πολλοὶ γὰρ
ἐξ αὐτῶν ἀπέθανον.

—Galen, *De alimentorum facultatibus* II.67
(VI.655–56K)

Coming to mushrooms: porcinis, when well boiled in water, come pretty close to being a completely bland food. But, of course, no one eats them plain like this; they prepare them and season them in all sorts of different ways, just as they do for all the other foods that people don't use for any particular quality. The nourishment that results from these mushrooms is phlegmy, obviously also cold, and, if you eat too much of them, unwholesome. In fact, these are the least harmful of the mushrooms; second after these are creminis. As for the rest, it is safer to just not touch them; many people have died from them.

—Galen, *On the Properties of Foodstuffs*

VEGETABLES AND LEGUMES

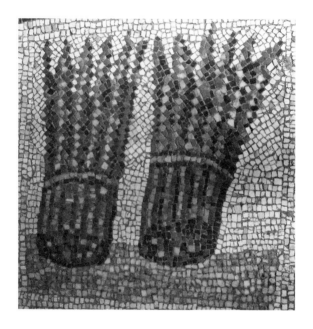

Lettuce

προύκριναν πολλοὶ τῶν ἰατρῶν τὸ λάχανον
τοῦτο τῶν ἄλλων ἁπάντων. . . . γιγνώσκειν
δὲ χρή, πάντων τῶν λαχάνων ὀλίγιστόν τε
καὶ κακόχυμον αἷμα γεννώντων, ἐκ τῆς θριδακίνης οὐ πολὺ μὲν οὐδὲ κακόχυμον, οὐ
μὴν εὔχυμόν γε τελέως αἷμα γίγνεσθαι.
ἐσθίουσι δ᾽ αὐτὴν ὡς τὰ πολλὰ μὲν ὠμήν·
ὅταν δ᾽ εἰς σπέρματος γένεσιν ἐξορμᾶν
ὑπάρξηται θέρους ὥρᾳ, προεψήσαντες ἐν
ὕδατι γλυκεῖ προσφέρονται δι᾽ ἐλαίου καὶ
γάρου καὶ ὄξους ἢ διά τινος τῶν ὑποτριμμά-
των, καὶ μάλισθ᾽ ὅσα διὰ τυροῦ σκευάζεται.
χρῶνται δ᾽ αὐτῇ καὶ πρὶν εἰς καυλὸν ἐξορ-
μῆσαι πολλοὶ δι᾽ ὕδατος ἕψοντες, ὥσπερ
κἀγὼ νῦν ἠρξάμην, ἀφ᾽ οὗ τῶν ὀδόντων
ἔχω φαύλως. εἰδὼς γάρ τις τῶν ἑταίρων ἐν
ἔθει μὲν ὂν ἐκ πολλοῦ μοι τὸ λάχανον, ἐπί-
πονον δὲ νῦν ἴσχοντι τὴν μάσησιν, εἰσηγή-
σατο τὴν ἕψησιν.

Lettuce

Many doctors prefer lettuce to all other vegetables.... One ought to be aware that all vegetables produce scant and unwholesome blood, but the blood resulting from lettuce, though not plentiful, is not unwholesome (though it is not completely wholesome either). People usually eat it raw; but whenever in the summer it starts to go to seed, they boil it in sweet water and serve it with oil, fish sauce, and vinegar or with one of the compound dressings, especially those prepared with cheese. Many people boil it in water even before it starts to sprout, just as I have now begun to do, ever since my teeth have been troubling me. For, one of my friends — knowing that this vegetable had long been a habit with me, but that I now found chewing difficult — suggested boiling.

ἐχρώμην δὲ θριδακίναις ἐν νεότητι μὲν ἐκ-
χολουμένης μοι συνεχῶς τῆς ἄνω γαστρὸς
ἐμψύξεως ἕνεκεν, ὁπότε δ' εἰς τὴν καθεστη-
κυῖαν ἡλικίαν ἦλθον, ἄκος ἦν μοι μόνον τὸ
λάχανον τοῦτο τῆς ἀγρυπνίας, ἔμπαλιν ἢ
ὡς ὅτε μειράκιον ἦν ἐσπουδακότι περὶ τὸν
ὕπνον. εἰθισμένος τε γὰρ ἑκουσίως ἀγρυ-
πνεῖν ἐπὶ νεότητος ἅμα τε καὶ τῆς τῶν παρακ-
μαζόντων ἡλικίας ἀγρυπνητικῆς οὔσης,
ἀκουσίως ἀγρυπνῶν ἐδυσφόρουν, καί μοι
μόνον ἀλεξιφάρμακον ἀγρυπνίας ἦν ἑσπέ-
ρας ἐσθιομένη θριδακίνη.

—Galen, *De alimentorum facultatibus* II.40
(VI.624–26K)

θριδακίνη μὲν οὖν καὶ τροφὴ καὶ φάρμακον
ψυχρόν.

—Galen, *De temperamentis* III.4 (I.681K)

When I was a young man and my upper stomach was constantly full of bile, I used to use lettuce for its cooling properties; but when I reached middle age, this vegetable was my go-to cure for insomnia, for at that age, contrary to my teenage years, I was serious about sleep. I used to make a habit of voluntarily staying up late when I was young, but insomnia is a natural part of aging, and I became very annoyed at being unable to sleep against my will; the only remedy against insomnia for me was lettuce eaten in the evening.

—Galen, *On the Properties of Foodstuffs*

Lettuce is both a food and a cooling drug.

—Galen, *On Mixtures*

θρίδαξ ἥμερος εὐστόμαχος, ὑποψύχουσα,
ὑπνωτική, κοιλίας μαλακτική, γάλακτος
κατασπαστική· ἑψηθεῖσα δὲ γίνεται τροφι-
μωτέρα, ἄπλυτος δὲ ἐσθιομένη στομαχι-
κοῖς ἁρμοζεῖ. . . . αὐταὶ δὲ συνεχῶς ἐσθιόμε-
ναι ἀμβλυωπίας εἰσὶ ποιητικαί· ταριχεύονται
δὲ ἐν ἅλμῃ.

—Dioscorides, *De materia medica* II.136

Lactucas:

Cum oxyporio et aceto et modico liquamine ad digestionem et inflationem et ne
lactucae ledant:

cumini uncias II
gengiber unciam I
rutae viridis unciam I
dactilorum pinguium scripulos XII
piperis unciam I

Cultivated lettuce is easy on the stomach, cooling, sleep-inducing, softening to the bowels, and stimulating for milk-production. When boiled, it is more nutritious; when eaten unwashed, it is helpful for people prone to stomach issues. . . . When eaten continuously it is productive of dim-sightedness. People pickle it in brine.

—Dioscorides, *Medical Substances*

Recipe for lettuce:

Serve with a piquant sauce, vinegar, or a little fish sauce to help with digestion and flatulence and to prevent the lettuce from doing any harm:

2 oz. cumin
1 oz. ginger
1 oz. fresh rue
½ oz. plump dates
1 oz. pepper

mellis uncias VIIII

(cuminum aut Aethiopicum aut Siriacum
aut Libicum)

Tundes cuminum et postea infundes in
aceto. Cum siccaverit postea melle omnia
conprehendes; cum necesse fuerit dimidium
coclearum <cum> aceto et liquamine modico
misces aut post cenam dimidium coclearum
accipies.

—*Apicius* III.18.2

Cabbage

κράμβη θερμαίνει καὶ διαχωρεῖ· χολώδεα
δε ἄγει.

—Hippocratic *De victu* II.54.5

Brassica est quae omnibus holeribus antistat.
Eam esto vel coctam vel crudam: crudam si

9 oz. honey
(the cumin should be Ethiopian, Syrian,
  or Libyan)

Grind the cumin and then pour it into
some vinegar. Once that has dried, mix
everything together with the honey. When
it is time to use it, mix half a scoopful with
vinegar and a little fish sauce; or you can
just eat half a scoopful after dinner.

—*Apicius' Cookbook*

Cabbage

Cabbage warms the body and passes
easily through the bowels; it carries off
bilious matter.

—Hippocratic *Regimen*

Cabbage is the vegetable that surpasses all
others. Eat it raw or cooked. If you eat it

edes, in acetum intinguito: mirifice concoquit, alvum bonam facit lotiumque ad omnes
res salubre est.

Si voles in convivio multum bibere cena-
reque libenter, ante cenam esto crudam
quantum voles ex aceto; et item, ubi ce-
naveris, comesto aliqua V folia: reddet te
quasi nihil ederis, bibesque quantum voles.

. . .

Et si voles eam consectam, lautam, siccam, sale, aceto sparsam esse, salubrius
nihil est. Quo libentius edis, aceto mulso
spargito—lautam, siccam et rutam, corian-
drum sectam sale sparsam paulo libentius
edes—, id bene faciet et mali nihil sinet in
corpore consistere et alvum bonam faciet;
si quid antea mali intus erit, omnia sana faciet

raw, sprinkle it with vinegar. It digests marvelously, does the belly good, and the resulting urine is a cure-all.

If you wish to drink a lot and gorge yourself at a party: before the dinner, eat as much raw cabbage as you want, dressed in vinegar, and then, when you have dined, eat about five leaves—it will make you as if you had eaten nothing and you will drink as much as you like.

. . .

If you like it chopped, washed, dried, salted, and sprinkled with vinegar, nothing is healthier. If you want to make it nicer to eat, sprinkle it with honeyed vinegar—it is even nicer to eat washed, dried, with chopped rue and cilantro, and sprinkled with salt—this does you good and allows nothing bad to remain in the body and does the bowels good. If there was something unhealthy inside before, it makes everything

et de capite et de oculis omnia deducet
et sanum faciet; hanc mane esse oportet
ieiunum.

. . .

Alvum deicere hoc modo oportet: si vis
bene tibi deicere, sume tibi ollam, addito eo
aquae sextarios sex et eo addito ungulam de
perna; si ungulam non habebis, addito de
perna frustum p. S quam minime pingue;
ubi iam coctum incipit esse, eo addito
brassicae coliculos duos, betae coliculos II
cum radice sua, feliculae pullum, herbae
mercurialis non multum, mitulorum L. II,
piscem capitonem et scorpionem I, cochleas
sex et lentis pugillum. Haec omnia decoquito
usque ad sextarios III iuris; oleum ne addi-
deris; indidem sume tibi sextarium unum
tepidum, adde vini Coi cyathum unum,
bibe, interquiesce; deinde iterum eodem
modo, deinde tertium: purgabis te bene.
Et si voles insuper vinum Coum mixtum

healthy and removes everything built up in the head and the eyes and makes them healthy. You ought to eat it in the morning before you eat anything else.

. . .

It is good to get the bowels moving in this way: if you wish to really cleanse yourself, get yourself a pot and add to it six pints of water and add to that the hoof from a leg of ham (if you don't have the hoof, add a ½ lb. piece of the leg, as lean as possible). When it begins to be cooked, add to it two small heads of cabbage, two small heads of beet (with root attached), a sprout of polypody fern, a little bit of mercury herb, 2 lbs. of mussels, a *capito* fish and a scorpion fish, six snails, and a fistful of lentils. Boil all this down until it is three pints of juice. Do not add oil. Take for yourself one pint warm from the pot, add one cyathus[1] of Coan wine, drink it, rest, then repeat in the same way, then repeat a

bibere, licebit bibas. Ex iis tot rebus quod scriptum est unum, quod eorum vis, alvum deicere potest; verum ea re tot res sunt, uti bene deicias, et suave est.

—Cato, *De agricultura* 156, 157.5–6, 158

καὶ ταύτην οἱ πολλοὶ μὲν ὡς ὄψον ἐσθίουσιν, ἰατροὶ δ' ὡς φαρμάκῳ ξηραίνοντι χρῶνται. . . . τὸν μὲν χυλὸν αὐτῆς ἔχειν τι καθαρτικόν, αὐτὸ δὲ τὸ σῶμα κατὰ τὸν τοῦ ξηραίνειν λόγον ἐπέχειν μᾶλλον ἢ προτρέπειν εἰς ὑποχώρησιν. . . . οὐ μὴν εὔχυμόν γ' ἐστὶν ἔδεσμα κράμβη, καθάπερ ἡ θρῖδαξ, ἀλλὰ καὶ μοχθηρὸν ἔχει καὶ δυσώδη τὸν χυλόν.

—Galen, *De alimentorum facultatibus* II.44 (VI.631K)

third time. You will purge yourself well. And if you wish to drink diluted Coan wine in addition, it is fine to drink it. Out of all the things that are mentioned here, any one that you pick is able to cleanse the bowels; there are so many things in this recipe because it really cleanses the bowels and it tastes good.

—Cato, *On Farming*

Most people eat cabbage as a relish, but doctors use it as a drying drug.... Its juice has a certain cleansing action, but the vegetable itself, because of its drying power, stops up the body more than it encourages it to evacuate the bowels.... Cabbage is emphatically not a wholesome food, like lettuce is, but has a pernicious and bad-smelling juice.

—Galen, *On the Properties of Foodstuffs*

Arugula

θερμαίνει σαφῶς πάνυ τοῦτο τὸ λάχανον,
ὥστ᾽ οὐδὲ μόνον ἐσθίειν αὐτὸ ῥάδιον ἄνευ
τοῦ μῖξαι τοῖς θύλλοις τῆς θριδακίνης, ἀλλὰ
καὶ σπέρμα γεννᾶν πεπίστευται καὶ τὰς
πρὸς συνουσίας ὁρμὰς ἐπεγείρειν. κεφαλ-
αλγὲς δ᾽ ἐστί, καὶ μᾶλλον ἐάν τις αὐτὸ μόνον
ἐσθίῃ.

—Galen, *De alimentorum facultatibus* II.52
(VI.639K)

εὔζωμον πλεῖον βρωθὲν συνουσίαν παρ-
ορμᾷ ... οὐρητικὸν ὑπάρχον καὶ πεπτικὸν
καὶ εὐκοίλιον· ... ἀποτίθενται δὲ αὐτὸ πρὸς
τὸ πλείονα μένειν χρόνον γάλακτι ἢ ὄξει
φυρῶντες καὶ ἀναπλάσσοντες τροχίσκους.

—Dioscorides, *De materia medica* II.140

Arugula

This vegetable is obviously extremely heating, so that it is not easy to eat it on its own without mixing it with some lettuce leaves, but it is also believed to promote the production of semen and to rouse desire for sex. It causes headaches, though, especially if you eat it on its own.

—Galen, *On the Properties of Foodstuffs*

Arugula eaten in large quantities stimulates the sex-drive; . . . it is diuretic, easy to digest, and good for the bowels. . . . To keep it good for a long time, people preserve it by mixing it up with milk or vinegar and rolling it into little wheels.

—Dioscorides, *Medical Substances*

Cucumbers

σίκυς ἥμερος εὐκοίλιος, εὐστόμαχος, ψυ-
κτικός, οὐ φθειρόμενος, κύστει ἁρμόδιος,
ἀνακτητικὸς λειποθυμιῶν ὀσφραινόμε-
νος. . . . ὁ δὲ χυλὸς σὺν τῷ σπέρματι μιγεὶς
ἀλεύρῳ καὶ ξηρανθεὶς ἐν ἡλίῳ σμῆγμα γίνεται ῥυπτικὸν καὶ προσώπου λαμπρυντικόν.

—Dioscorides, *De materia medica* II.135

πέττουσι δ᾽ αὐτοὺς ἔνιοι, καθάπερ καὶ ἄλλα
τινὰ τῶν τοῖς πολλοῖς ἀπεπτουμένων, οἰκει-
ότητι τῆς πρὸς αὐτὰ φύσεως . . . τοῖς οὖν
τοὺς σικύους καλῶς πέττουσιν, ὅταν αὐτῷ
τούτῳ θαρσήσαντες ἄδην αὐτῶν ἐμφορη-
θῶσι, χρόνῳ πολλῷ ψυχρὸν καὶ μετρίως
παχὺν ἀθροίζεσθαι συμβαίνει κατὰ τὰς
φλέβας χυμόν, οὐκ εὐπετῶς ἐπιδέξασθαι
δυνάμενον τὴν εἰς αἷμα χρηστὸν ἀλλοίωσιν

Cucumbers

The cucumber is easy on the bowels and the stomach, cooling, in no way harmful, good for the bladder, and revivifying for the fainted if they smell it. . . . The juice and seeds, when mixed with whole meal flour and dried out in the sun, make a soap that is cleansing and leaves the face glowing.

—Dioscorides, *Medical Substances*

Some people are able to digest these (just like there are those who can digest other foods that are indigestible to most people) because their nature is similar to them. . . . But even those who digest cucumbers well, when they get overconfident in this ability and gorge themselves on them, eventually find that a cold and fairly thick humor collects in their veins, since it is not

ἐν τῇ κατὰ τὰς φλέβας πέψει. πάντων οὖν
διὰ τοῦτ᾽ ἀπέχεσθαι συμβουλεύω τῶν κα-
κοχύμων ἐδεσμάτων, κἂν εὔπεπτά τισιν ᾖ.

—Galen, *De alimentorum facultatibus* II.6
(VI.567, 569)

Cartilaginum generis extraque terram est
cucumis, mira voluptate Tiberio principi
expetitus; nullo quippe non die contigit ei,
pensiles eorum hortos promoventibus in
solem rotis olitoribus rursusque hibernis
diebus intra specularium munimenta revo-
cantibus. . . . Vivunt hausti in stomacho in

amenable to easily undergoing the trans-
formation into useful blood in the final
stage of digestion in the veins. For this reason, I advise people to avoid all unwholesome foods, even if they are easily digestible
to some.

—Galen, *On the Properties of Foodstuffs*

The cucumber is a fleshy type of vegetable
that grows above the ground. The Emperor Tiberius had a remarkable passion
for them. On no day were they not available to him: his gardeners had moveable
beds of them, which they rolled on wheels
into the sun, and on winter days they
brought them back under glass-paned
frames. . . . Once swallowed, cucumbers
dwell in the stomach into the following
day, and are not able to be digested with

posterum diem nec perfici queunt in cibis, non insalubres tamen plurimum.

—Pliny the Elder, *Naturalis historia* XIX.23.64–65

Onions

κρόμμυον τῇ μὲν ὄψει ἀγαθόν, τῷ δὲ σώματι κακόν, διότι θερμὸν καὶ καυσῶδες καὶ οὐ διαχωρεῖ· τροφὴν μὲν γὰρ οὐ δίδωσι τῷ σώματι οὐδὲ ὠφελίην· θερμαῖνον δὲ ξηραίνει διὰ τὸν ὀπόν.

—Hippocratic *De victu* II.54.1

κρόμυον· δριμύτερον τὸ μακρὸν τοῦ στρογγύλου καὶ τὸ ξανθὸν τοῦ λευκοῦ καὶ τὸ ξηρὸν τοῦ χλωροῦ καὶ τὸ ὠμὸν τοῦ ὀπτοῦ καὶ ταριχηροῦ. ἔστι δὲ ἄπαντα δηκτικὰ καὶ πνευματωτικά, ὀρέξεως ἐκκλητικά, λεπτυντικά, διψώδη, ἀσώδη, ἀποκαθαρτικά,

the rest of the food; they are not extremely unhealthy though.

—Pliny the Elder, *Natural History*

Onions

The onion is good for the vision, but bad for the body because it is hot and caustic and difficult to excrete; it does not give much nourishment or benefit to the body, but heats and dries it out because of its juice.

—Hippocratic *Regimen*

Onions: a scallion is more pungent than a round onion, a yellow one than a white, a dried one than a fresh, a raw one than a cooked or pickled one. All of them are sharp, productive of flatulence, stimulating to the appetite, thinning, thirst-making,

εὐκοίλια . . . σὺν ὀρνιθείῳ δὲ στέατι πρὸς
ἐκτρίμματα ὑποδημάτων χρήσιμος καὶ πρὸς
δυσηκοίαν καὶ συριγμοὺς καὶ πυρροοῦντα
ὦτα ὁ χυλὸς καὶ ὕδατος <ἐν>απολήμψεις,
καὶ πρὸς ἀλωπεκίας παρατριβόμενος.

—Dioscorides, *De materia medica* II.151

Lentils

ἀεὶ μὲν ὑγιεινότερα σώματι τὰ εὐτελέστ-
ερα . . . αὐτὸς δέ τις ἑαυτῷ παρακελευέσθω
μὴ πρὸ φακῆς λοπάδ᾽ αὔξων αἰεὶ μηδὲ πά-
ντως ὑπερβαίνων τὴν καρδαμίδα καὶ τὴν
ἐλαίαν ἐπὶ τὸ θρῖον καὶ τὸν ἰχθὺν εἰς στάσιν
ἐκ πλησμονῆς τὸ σῶμα καὶ ταραχὰς ἐμβάλ-
λειν καὶ διαρροίας.

—Plutarch, *De tuenda sanitate praecepta*
123d, 125f

nauseating, cleansing, easy on the bowels. . . .
Mixed with chicken fat, the juice is useful
for blisters caused by shoes, for difficulty
hearing, tinnitus, supporating ears, and
water in the ears, and for bald spots, if
you rub it on.

—Dioscorides, *Medical Substances*

Lentils

Less expensive things are always healthier
for the body. . . . Everyone should exhort
themselves not to forever be expanding
their dinner menu beyond lentils and especially not, by venturing beyond even
pepperwort and olives into little cakes and
fish, to throw their bodies into revolt—
upset stomachs and diarrhea!—through
overindulgence.

—Plutarch, *On Keeping Well*

φακοὶ καυσώδεις καὶ ταρακτικοί, οὔτε δια-
χωρέουσιν οὔτε ἱστᾶσιν.

—Hippocratic *De victu* II.45.2

φακὸς βιβρωσκόμενος συνεχῶς ἀμβλυω-
πός, δύσπεπτος, κακοστόμαχος, πνευμα-
τωτικὸς στομάχου καὶ ἐντέρων, κοιλίας τε
σταλτικὸς σὺν τῷ λέπει ἑψόμενος· διαφέ-
ρει δὲ αὐτοῦ ὁ ἑψανὸς καὶ μηδὲν ἀνιεὶς ἐν
τῇ βροχῇ μέλαν. δύναμιν δὲ ἔχει στυπτικήν,
ὅθεν κοιλίαν ἵστησι προαπολεπισθεὶς καὶ
ἑψηθεὶς ἐπιμελῶς, τοῦ πρώτου ἐν τῷ ἀφέ-
ψεσθαι ὕδατος ἀποχεομένου· λυτικὸν γὰρ
κοιλίας τὸ ἀφέψημα αὐτοῦ. ἔστι δὲ δυσόνειρος, ἄθετος πρὸς τὰ νευρώδη καὶ πνεύμονα καὶ κεφαλήν.

—Dioscorides, *De materia medica* II.107

Lentils are heating and disturbing; they neither pass through easily nor cause constipation.

—Hippocratic *Regimen*

The lentil, when eaten steadily, causes dim-sightedness, poor digestion, stomachache, gas in the stomach and intestines, and constipation of the bowels (when boiled with its husk). Boiled lentils that leave no blackness in the broth are preferable. They have a binding quality, which is why they cause the bowels to stop up when they are hulled and carefully boiled, with the first cooking water changed out (this cooking water is laxative to the bowels). They give bad dreams and are not helpful for the nerves, the lungs, or the head.

—Dioscorides, *Medical Substances*

εἰκότως οὖν οἱ πλεονάζοντες ἐν τούτῳ τῷ
ἐδέσματι τούς τε καλουμένους ἐλέφαντας
ἴσχουσι καὶ καρκίνους· ἐπιτήδειον γάρ ἐστι
τὸ παχὺ καὶ ξηρὸν ἔδεσμα μελαγχολικὸν
γεννᾶν χυμόν. οἷς οὖν ἐστιν ὑδατώδης τις
ἐν ταῖς σαρξὶ καχεξία, τούτοις μόνοις ὠφέ-
λιμον ἔδεσμα φακῆ, καθάπερ τοῖς ξηροῖς
καὶ αὐχμώδεσι βλαβερώτατον. ὡσαύτως δὲ
καὶ τὴν ὄψιν ἀμβλύνει μὲν τὴν ὑγιεινῶς δια-
κειμένην ὑπερξηραίνουσα, τὴν δ᾽ ἐναντίως
ἔχουσαν ὀνίνησιν.

—Galen, *De alimentorum facultatibus* I.18
(VI.526K)

Invenio apud auctores aequanimitatem fieri
vescentibus ea.

—Pliny the Elder, *Naturalis historia*
XVIII.31.123

People who overindulge in this food are likely to contract cancers and the disease known as elephantiasis; for a thick and dry food is inclined to produce black bile. Therefore, lentils are only a wholesome food for people whose flesh contains some imbalance toward moisture, and they are very harmful to dry and leathery people. In the same way, because they are excessively drying, they dull the sight in people whose vision is healthy, but they improve it in people whose vision is too moist.

—Galen, *On the Properties of Foodstuffs*

I find it written in authoritative sources that eating these makes you good-tempered.

—Pliny the Elder, *Natural History*

Beans

κύαμοι τρόφιμον καὶ στατικὸν καὶ φυσῶδες.

—Hippocratic *De victu* II.45.1

κύαμος Ἑλληνικὸς πνευματωτικός, φυσώ-
δης, δύσπεπτος, δυσόνειρος, βηχὶ δὲ σύμ-
φορος καὶ σαρκῶν γεννητικός . . . γίνεται
δὲ ἀφυσότερος τοῦ πρώτου ὕδατος κατὰ
τὴν ἕψησιν ἀποχεομένου.

—Dioscorides, *De materia medica* II.105

καὶ πλείστῳ γε τούτῳ τῷ ἐδέσματι καθ᾽ ἑκάστην ἡμέραν οἱ παρ᾽ ἡμῖν μονομάχοι χρῶνται, σαρκοῦντι τὴν τοῦ σώματος ἕξιν, οὐκ
ἐσφιγμένῃ καὶ πυκνῇ σαρκί, καθάπερ τὸ χοί-
ρειον κρέας, ἀλλὰ χαυνοτέρᾳ πως μᾶλλον.
φυσῶδες δ᾽ ἐστὶν ἔδεσμα, κἂν ἐπὶ πλεῖστον

Beans

Beans are nourishing, binding, and flatulent.

—Hippocratic *Regimen*

The fava bean is full of wind, flatulent, difficult to digest, and it causes bad dreams; but it is helpful for a cough and bulks people up.... It becomes less flatulent if you change out the first water when you boil it.

—Dioscorides, *Medical Substances*

My gladiators[2] eat a great deal of this food every day; it puts flesh on their bodies, but not a firm and thick flesh, like pork does, but one that is somehow flabbier. It is a flatulent food, even if well boiled (really, no matter how it is prepared)....

ἑψηθῇ κἂν ὁπωσοῦν σκευασθῇ.... τοῖς δὲ προσέχουσι τὸν νοῦν καὶ παρακολουθοῦσι ταῖς ἑπομέναις ἑκάστῳ τῶν ἐδεσμάτων δια-θέσεσιν αἴσθησις γίγνεται καθ᾽ ὅλον τὸ σῶμα τάσεώς τινος ὡς ὑπὸ πνεύματος φυ-σώδους, καὶ μάλισθ᾽ ὅταν ἀήθης τις ᾖ τοῦδε τοῦ βρώματος ἢ μὴ καλῶς ἡψημένον προσε-νέγκηται.... οὐ μόνον δ᾽ ὠμοὺς ἐσθίουσιν τοὺς χλωροὺς κυάμους οἱ πολλοὶ τῶν ἀν-θρώπων, ἀλλὰ καὶ μετὰ κρεῶν χοιρείων ἕψοντες, ὥσπερ τὰ λάχανα, κατὰ δὲ τοὺς ἀγροὺς καὶ μετ᾽ αἰγείων τε καὶ προβατείων. ᾐσθημένοι δ᾽ αὐτῶν τοῦ φυσώδους οἱ ἄν-θρωποι μιγνύουσι κρομύων, ὅταν ἐν λοπάδι σκευάζωσιν ἐξ αὐτῶν ἔτνος. ἔνιοι δὲ καὶ χωρὶς τοῦ συνέψειν ὠμὰ τὰ κρόμυα προσφέ-ρονται μετ᾽ αὐτοῦ. τὸ γὰρ τοι φυσῶδες ἐν ἅπασι τοῖς ἐδέσμασιν ὑπὸ τῶν θερμαινό-ντων τε καὶ λεπτυνόντων ἐπανορθοῦται.

—Galen, *De alimentorum facultatibus* I.19 (VI.529–32K)

People who pay attention and keep track of the sensations that follow each of the foods they eat will notice a certain tension throughout their whole body, as if it is inflated by wind, and especially so if someone is unaccustomed to this food or if they are served some that was not cooked well. . . . Most people eat fava beans either raw and green or boiled with pork, just like vegetables; in the country, they also eat them with lamb and beef. Having observed how flatulent they are, people mix in onions whenever they make a dish of bean stew. Some people even add raw onions to them without boiling them together. Certainly, flatulence in any food is counteracted by means of warming and thinning things.

—Galen, *On the Properties of Foodstuffs*

Wheaten Breads

Tritici genera plura quae fecere gentes. Italico nullum equidem comparaverim candore ac pondere, quo maxime discernitur. . . . Siliginem proprie dixerim tritici delicias sive candore esse sive virtute sive

GRAINS

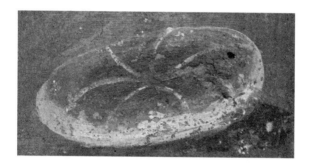

Wheaten Breads

There are many varieties of wheat, which different peoples cultivate. I would say that none is comparable to the Italian variety in terms of whiteness and weight, for which it has the highest renown. . . . I think I can accurately say that Italian soft wheat is the sweetheart of the wheat

pondere.... E siligine lautissimus panis pistrinarumque opera laudatissima.

—Pliny the Elder, *Naturalis historia* XVIII.12.63, 20.85–86

καὶ παρά γε τοῖς Ῥωμαίοις, ὥσπερ οὖν καὶ παρὰ τοῖς ἄλλοις σχεδὸν ἅπασιν, ὧν ἄρχουσιν, ὁ μὲν καθαρώτατος ἄρτος ὀνομάζεται σιλιγνίτης, ὁ δ' ἐφεξῆς αὐτῷ σεμιδαλίτης.... τροφιμώτατος μὲν οὖν ἐστιν ὁ σιλιγνίτης ἄρτος, ἐφεξῆς δ' ὁ σεμιδαλίτης, καὶ τρίτος ὁ μέσος τε καὶ συγκομιστός· ἐφ' ᾧ τέταρτόν ἐστι τὸ τῶν ῥυπαρῶν εἶδος, ὧν ἔσχατος ὁ πιτυρίας, ὃς δὴ καὶ ἀτροφώτατός ἐστι καὶ μάλιστα τῶν ἄλλων ὑπέρχεται κατὰ γαστέρα....

family, whether judged by whiteness, wholesomeness, or weight. . . . From soft wheat come both the most refined bread and the best-rated confections of pastry shops.

—Pliny the Elder, *Natural History*

Among the Romans (and likewise, therefore, among just about all the other peoples whom they rule), the purest bread is called soft wheat, and the next best fine wheat. . . . Soft wheat is the most nourishing bread, and fine wheat is next best; in third place is medium-processed whole wheat; and after that, in fourth place, is the kind that looks like the wheat has not been processed at all, the worst of which is bran bread, which is least nourishing and passes most vigorously of all the breads down through the stomach. . . .

ἄριστος μὲν οὖν ἄρτος εἰς ὑγίειάν ἐστιν
ἀνθρώπῳ μήτε νέῳ μήτε γυμναζομένῳ ὁ
πλεῖστον μὲν ζύμης ἔχων, πλεῖστον δ' ἁλῶν,
ἐπὶ πλεῖστον δ' ὑπὸ τοῦ τεχνίτου πρὶν ὀπτᾶ-
σθαι κατειργασμένος, ὠπτημένος δ' ἐν κρι-
βάνῳ συμμέτρως θερμῷ. . . . κρίσις δὲ τοῦ
πλείστου κατὰ τὴν ζύμην καὶ τοὺς ἅλας ἡ
γεῦσις ἔστω σοι· τὸ γὰρ ἤδη λυποῦν ἐν τῇ
τούτων πλείονι μίξει μοχθηρόν. εἰς ὅσον οὖν
ἡ γεῦσις οὐδέπω γνωρίζει τὴν ἐκ τῆς μίξεως
ἀηδίαν, εἰς τοσοῦτον βέλτιόν ἐστιν αὐξάνειν
αὐτῶν τὸ πλῆθος.

ὅσοι δὲ τὸν πλυτὸν ἄρτον ἐπενόησαν
σκευάζειν, ἀτροφώτερον μὲν εὖρον ἔδεσμα, πεφευγὸς δ' ὡς οἷόν τε μάλιστα τὴν ἐκ
τῆς ἐμφράξεως βλάβην. ἥκιστα γὰρ ὁ ἄρτος
οὗτος ἔχει τὸ παχὺ καὶ γλίσχρον ἀερωδέ-
στερος ἀντὶ γεωδεστέρου γεγονός. ὁρᾶται

So, the best bread in terms of healthfulness (for a person who is neither young nor in athletic training) is the one with the most amount of leavening, with the most amount of salt, which received the most thorough kneading by its maker before it was baked, and which was baked in a moderately hot oven. . . . Let taste be your guide to the upper limit when it comes to leavening and salt: for if the preponderance of one of these makes the bread unpleasant, that is pernicious. Basically, it is better to increase the quantity of each of these up to the threshold at which taste does not yet register anything unpleasant in the mixture.

Whoever contrives to prepare refined bread finds that, while it is not a terribly nourishing food, it avoids to the greatest degree possible the harm that comes from impaction. For this type of bread is the farthest from being thick and sticky — it is

δ' ἡ κουφότης αὐτοῦ διά τε τοῦ σταθμοῦ
κἀκ τοῦ μὴ δύεσθαι καθ' ὕδατος, ἀλλ' ἐπ-
οχεῖσθαι τρόπον φελλοῦ.

—Galen, *De alimentorum facultatibus* I.2,
4–5 (VI.483–84, 494K)

Barley

κριθαὶ φύσει μὲν ὑγρὸν καὶ ψυχρόν. ἔνι δὲ
καὶ καθαρτικόν τι ἀπὸ τοῦ χυλοῦ τοῦ
ἀχύρου. . . . ὅταν δὲ πυρωθέωσι, τὸ μὲν
ὑγρὸν καὶ καθαρτικὸν ὑπὸ τοῦ πυρὸς οἴχε-
ται, τὸ δὲ καταλειπόμενον ψυχρὸν καὶ
ξηρόν. ὅσα οὖν δεῖ ψῦξαι καὶ ξηρῆναι, ἄλφιτον διαπρήσσεται ὧδε χρεωμένῳ μάζῃ
παντοδαπῇ. δύναμιν δὲ ἔχει ἡ μᾶζα τοιήνδε.
τὰ συγκομιστὰ ἄλευρα τροφὴν μὲν ἔχει

more airy than solid. Its sponginess is evident from its weight and from the fact that it does not sink in the water but floats like a cork.

—Galen, *On the Properties of Foodstuffs*

Barley

Barley is naturally moist and cold; but it also has a sort of purgative quality from the juice of its chaff. . . . When it is toasted, the moist and purgative part is removed by the fire, and what remains is cold and dry. Therefore, whenever there is a need to cool and to dry, barley meal will accomplish it, if you make it into any sort of barley cake: that is the sort of power that barley cakes have. Unhulled barley is less nutritious but passes through the bowels more easily; pearled

ἐλάσσω, διαχωρεῖ δὲ μᾶλλον· τὰ δὲ καθαρὰ
τροφιμώτερα, ἧσσον δὲ διαχωρεῖ.

—Hippocratic *De victu* II.40.1–2

οἱ παλαιοὶ δὲ καὶ τοῖς στρατευομένοις ἄλ-
φιτα παρεσκεύαζον. ἀλλ᾽ οὐ τό γε νῦν ἔτι
τὸ Ῥωμαίων στρατιωτικὸν ἀλφίτοις χρῆται
κατεγνωκὸς αὐτῶν ἀσθένειαν. ὀλίγην γὰρ
τροφὴν δίδωσι τοῖς σώμασι.

—Galen, *De alimentorum facultatibus* I.11
(VI.507K)

Oats

τροφὴ δ᾽ ἐστὶν ὑποζυγίων, οὐκ ἀνθρώπων.

—Galen, *De alimentorum facultatibus* I.14
(VI.522–23K)

barley is more nutritious but passes less easily.

—Hippocratic *Regimen*

The ancients provided barley even to their soldiers. But in modern times the Roman military no longer uses barley, condemning it on the grounds that it weakens them. For it provides little nourishment to the body.

—Galen, *On the Properties of Foodstuffs*

Oats

This is food for beasts of burden, not for people.

—Galen, *On the Properties of Foodstuffs*

GRAINS

Rice

τούτῳ τῷ σπέρματι πάντες εἰς ἐπίσχεσιν
γαστρὸς χρῶνται τὴν ἕψησιν αὐτοῦ παρα-
πλησίαν ποιούμενοι χόνδρῳ. δυσπεπτότε-
ρον δ᾽ ἐστὶ χόνδρου καὶ τρέφον ἧττον,
ὥσπερ γε καὶ εἰς ἐδωδῆς ἡδονὴν ἀπολειπό-
μενον αὐτοῦ πάμπολυ.

—Galen, *De alimentorum facultatibus* I.17
(VI.525K)

Rice

Everyone uses this grain to settle the stomach, preparing it in a way very similar to cream of wheat. But it is harder to digest and less nourishing than cream of wheat, and also just generally less pleasurable to eat.

—Galen, *On the Properties of Foodstuffs*

DAIRY

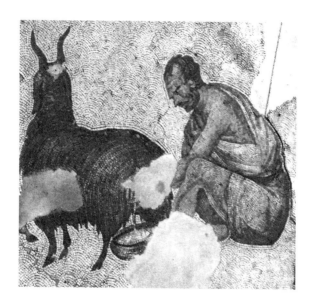

DAIRY

Milk

διαφέρον μὲν καὶ κατὰ τὰς ὥρας τοῦ ἔτους
οὐ σμικρὰν διαφοράν, ἔτι δὲ μείζω τὴν
κατ᾽ αὐτὰ τὰ ζῷα. τὸ μὲν γὰρ τῶν βοῶν
παχύτατόν τ᾽ ἐστὶ καὶ λιπαρώτατον, ὑγρότατον δὲ καὶ ἥκιστα λιπαρὸν τὸ τῆς καμή-
λου καὶ μετὰ ταύτην ἵππου, μετὰ δὲ ταύτην
ὄνου· σύμμετρον δὲ τῇ συστάσει τὸ τῆς
αἰγός ἐστι γάλα· τὸ δὲ τοῦ προβάτου παχύτερον τούτου. κατὰ δὲ τὰς ὥρας τοῦ
ἔτους ὑγρότατον μέν ἐστι τὸ μετὰ τὴν ἀπο-
κύησιν, ἀεὶ δὲ καὶ μᾶλλον ἐν τῷ προϊέναι
παχύνεται. καὶ κατὰ μέσον τὸ θέρος ἐν τῷ
μέσῳ καὶ αὐτὸ τῆς ἑαυτοῦ φύσεως καθί-
σταται. μετὰ δὲ τὸν καιρὸν τοῦτον ἤδη παχύνεται κατὰ βραχύ, μέχριπερ ἂν παύση-
ται τελέως. ἔστι δ᾽ ὥσπερ ὑγρότατον ἦρος,
οὕτω καὶ πλεῖστον. . . .

εὐχυμότατον εἶναι τὸ ἄριστον γάλα
σχεδὸν ἁπάντων, ὅσα προσφερόμεθα. μὴ

Milk

Milk differs from season to season in no small degree, but it differs even more depending on which animal it comes from. Cow's milk is the thickest and fattiest; the most liquid and least fatty milk is that from camels, next is horse's milk, and after that the one from donkeys. Goat's milk is intermediate in its composition, while sheep's milk is a little thicker. As far as the seasons of the year, it is most liquid after the spring birthing season and progressively thickens as time passes from that; at the midpoint of summer it, too, is at the midpoint of its nature. From that point onward, it thickens little by little until it dries up altogether. Just as it is most liquid in the spring, it is also most abundant then. . . .

The best milk is just about the most wholesome of all the foods that we consume.

παρακούσῃς δὲ τοῦ προσκειμένου κατὰ τὸν λόγον! οὐ γὰρ ἁπλῶς εἶπον εὐχυμότατον εἶναι γάλα πᾶν, ἀλλὰ προσέθηκα τὸ ἄριστον. ὡς τό γε κακόχυμον γάλα τοσούτου δεῖ συντελεῖν εἰς εὐχυμίαν, ὥστε καὶ τοὺς εὐχύμους χρωμένους αὐτῷ κακοχύμους ἐργάζεται.

—Galen, *De alimentorum facultatibus* III.14 (VI.681–82, 685K)

Cheeses

τυρὸς ἰσχυρὸν καὶ καυσῶδες καὶ τρόφιμον καὶ στάσιμον· ἰσχυρὸν μέν, ὅτι ἔγγιστα γενέσιός ἐστι, τρόφιμον δέ, ὅτι τοῦ γάλακτος τὸ σαρκῶδές ἐστιν ὑπόλοιπον, καυσῶδες δέ, ὅτι λιπαρόν, στάσιμον δέ, ὅτι ὀπῷ καὶ πυτίῃ συνέστηκεν.

—Hippocratic *De victu* II.51

But don't be careless about reading the nuances of my words! For I did not say unequivocally that all milk is the most wholesome, but added the word "best." Poor-quality milk is so far from being wholesome that it makes even healthily balanced people who drink it have unhealthy humors.

—Galen, *On the Properties of Foodstuffs*

Cheeses

Cheese is strong, heating, nourishing, and constipating: strong because it is closely akin to creating life; nourishing because the solid part of milk remains in it; heating because it is fatty; constipating because it is solidified by means of fig-juice or rennet.

—Hippocratic *Regimen*

παμπόλλης δ᾽ οὔσης κατὰ μέρος ἐν αὐτοῖς διαφορᾶς κατά τε τὰς φύσεις τῶν ζῴων καὶ τοὺς τρόπους τῆς σκευασίας καὶ προσέτι τὰς ἡλικίας αὐτῶν τῶν τυρῶν, ἐγὼ πειράσομαι κἀνταῦθα περιορίσαι τὴν δύναμιν αὐτῶν ὀλίγοις σκοποῖς, οἷς προσέχων τις ἐκ τοῦ ῥᾴστου διαγνώσεται τὸν ἀμείνω τε καὶ χείρω. κατὰ γένος μὲν οὖν οἱ σκοποὶ διττοὶ τυγχάνουσιν ὄντες, ὁ μὲν ἕτερος ἐν τῇ ποιᾷ συστάσει τῆς οὐσίας τοῦ τυροῦ, καθ᾽ ἣν μαλακώτερος ἢ σκληρότερος γίγνεται καὶ πυκνότερος ἢ χαυνότερος καὶ κολλωδέστερος ἢ ψαθυρώτερος, ὁ δ᾽ ἕτερος ἐν τῇ γεύσει, καθ᾽ ἣν ἔν τισι μὲν αὐτῶν ὀξύτης ἐπικρατεῖ, κατ᾽ ἄλλους δὲ δριμύτης ἢ λιπαρότης ἢ γλυκύτης ἤ τινα τούτων ἢ οἷον ἰσομοιρία πάντων.

κατὰ δὲ τὰς ἐν εἴδει διαφορὰς τῶν εἰρημένων γενῶν ὁ μὲν μαλακώτερος τοῦ

There is enormous difference from cheese to cheese, in terms of the nature of the animals they derive from, the manner of their preparation, and, further, the age of the individual cheeses themselves. Nevertheless, I shall attempt here to overview their powers with a few things to look for: if you pay attention to these, you will easily be able to distinguish the better from the worse. In terms of type, there happen to be two things to look for. The first has to do with what sort of consistency the substance of the cheese has: so, softer or harder, denser or spongier, more glutinous or more crumbly. The second has to do with taste: so, in some a sharpness is dominant, in others a funkiness or a fattiness or a sweetness, either just one of these or a sort of equal combination of them all.

As for the differences in appearance: of the types just mentioned, the softer cheese

σκληροτέρου βελτίων, ὁ δ᾽ ἀραιὸς καὶ χαῦνος τοῦ πάνυ πυκνοῦ καὶ πεπιλημένου. μοχθηρῶν δ᾽ ὄντων τοῦ τε κολλώδους ἱκανῶς καὶ τοῦ ψαθυροῦ μέχρι τραχύτητος ὁ μέσος αὐτῶν ἐστι βελτίων.

κατὰ δὲ τὴν ἐν τῇ γεύσει διάγνωσιν ἁπάντων μὲν ἄριστος ὁ μηδε μίαν ἰσχυρὰν ἔχων ποιότητα, βραχὺ δέ τι τῶν ἄλλων ὑπερέχουσαν τὴν γλυκύτητα, βελτίων δὲ καὶ ὁ ἡδίων τοῦ ἀηδοῦς καὶ ὁ συμμέτρως ἁλῶν ἔχων τοῦ παμπόλλους ἢ μηδ᾽ ὅλως ἔχοντος. μετά γε μὴν τὸ προσενέγκασθαι τὸν οὕτω κριθέντα καὶ διὰ τῆς ἐρυγῆς ἔνεστι γνωρίζειν, ὁποῖος αὐτῶν ἐστιν ἀμείνων τε καὶ χείρων. ὁ μὲν γὰρ κατὰ βραχὺ μαραινομένην ἴσχων τὴν ποιότητα βελτίων, ὁ δὲ παραμένουσαν οὐκ ἀγαθός· εὔδηλος γὰρ οὗτός

is better than the harder one, the loosely textured and spongy better than the very dense and compressed. Both the noticeably glutinous cheese and the one that is crumbly to the point of roughness are pernicious, so the one at the midpoint between these two is better.

As for the differentiation in taste, the best of all is the one that has no single strong quality, but has sweetness dominating the others by some small amount; further, the pleasant cheese is better than the distasteful one, and the one with a moderate amount of salt is better than one with too much or one without any at all. Furthermore, even after someone who has chosen along these guidelines has eaten a cheese, it is possible for them to gather further information about the degree to which it is better or worse than the others by means of their belches: the one that has a quality to it that gradually fades

ἐστι δυσμετάβλητός τε καὶ δυσαλλοίωτος
ὤν, ὥστε καὶ δύσπεπτος.

—Galen, *De alimentorum facultatibus* III.16
(VI.697–99K)

Laus caseo Romae, ubi omnium gentium
bona comminus iudicantur, e provinciis
Nemausensi praecipua, e Lesure Gabali-
coque pagis; sed brevis ac musteo tantum
commendatio.

—Pliny the Elder, *Naturalis historia*
XI.97.240

away is better, but the one that lingers is not good (for this cheese is evidently difficult to alter and to change, with the result that it is also difficult to digest).

—Galen, *On the Properties of Foodstuffs*

At Rome (where the prime exports of all nations are judged directly against each other) the highest praise goes to the cheese from the territories around Nîmes, from the districts of Lozère and Gévaudan— though this commendation stands only for a short while, when the cheese is fresh.

—Pliny the Elder, *Natural History*

DAIRY

Butter

μετέχει δὲ πρὸς τοῖσδε καὶ τρίτου τοῦ λιπαροῦ χυμοῦ, πλείστου μέν, ὡς εἴρηται, τὸ τῶν βοῶν γάλα. διὸ καὶ σκευάζουσιν ἐξ αὐτοῦ τὸ καλούμενον βούτυρον, ὃ καὶ γευσάμενος καὶ θεασάμενος μόνον ἐναργῶς γνώσῃ, πόσον αὐτῷ λιπαρότητος μέτεστιν. εἰ δὲ καὶ χρίσας τι μέρος τοῦ σώματος ἀνατρίψαις αὐτό, λιπαινόμενον ὡς ἐξ ἐλαίου θεάσῃ τὸ δέρμα. . . . καὶ μέντοι καὶ οἱ ἄνθρωποι κατὰ πολλὰ τῶν ψυχρῶν χωρίων, ἐν οἷς ἀποροῦσιν ἐλαίου, χρῶνται λουόμενοι τῷ βουτύρῳ.

—Galen, *De alimentorum facultatibus* III.14 (VI.683–84K)

Butter

In addition to these two elements (curds and whey), milk also contains a third, fatty substance—cow's milk especially, as I have mentioned. And for this reason they also make from milk the substance known as butter: just from tasting and touching this it would immediately become obvious to you how much fat there is in it. Also, if you rub it on any part of your body as a moisturizer, you will observe that the skin glistens just like it would with olive oil. . . . In fact, people who inhabit many of the colder regions in which they lack olive oil use butter when they wash themselves.

—Galen, *On the Properties of Foodstuffs*

E lacte fit et butyrum, barbararum gentium lautissimus cibus et qui divites a plebe discernat, plurimum e bubulo, et inde nomen, pinguissimum ex ovillo—fit et ex caprino ... Quo magis virus resipit hoc praestantius iudicatur. . . . Natura eius adstringere, mollire, replere, purgare.

—Pliny the Elder, *Naturalis historia*
XXVIII.35.133–34

From milk is also made butter, a food highly prized by barbarian peoples for whom it distinguishes the rich from the poor; it is mostly made from cow's milk (hence the name), but the fattiest kind is from sheep's milk and it is also made from goat's milk. . . . The stronger a flavor it has, the more it is judged to be superior. . . . Its nature is to bind the bowels, make things supple, satiate, and cleanse.

—Pliny the Elder, *Natural History*

MEAT, POULTRY, AND EGGS

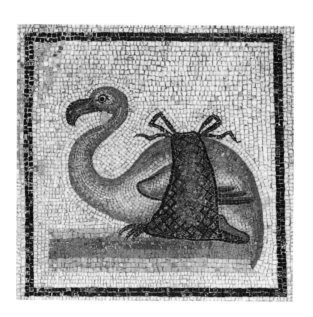

Pork

πάντων μὲν οὖν ἐδεσμάτων ἡ σὰρξ τῶν
ὑῶν ἐστι τροφιμωτάτη. καὶ τούτου πεῖραν
ἐναργεστάτην οἱ ἀθλοῦντες ἴσχουσιν. ἐπὶ
γὰρ τοῖς ἴσοις γυμνασίοις ἑτέρας τροφῆς
ἴσον ὄγκον ἐν ἡμέρᾳ μιᾷ προσενεγκάμενοι
κατὰ τὴν ὑστεραίαν εὐθέως ἀσθενέστεροι
γίγνονται· πλείοσι δ' ἐφεξῆς ἡμέραις τοῦτο
πράξαντες οὐκ ἀσθενέστεροι μόνον, ἀλλὰ
καὶ ἀτροφώτεροι σαφῶς φαίνονται. . . .
τῆς δ' ὑείας σαρκὸς τὴν πρὸς ἄνθρωπον
ὁμοιότητα καταμαθεῖν ἔστι κἀκ τοῦ τινας
ἐδηδοκότας ἀνθρωπείων κρεῶν ὡς ὑείων
οὐδεμίαν ὑπόνοιαν ἐσχηκέναι κατά τε τὴν
γεῦσιν αὐτῶν καὶ τὴν ὀσμήν· ἐφωράθη γὰρ
ἤδη που τοῦτο γεγονὸς ὑπό τε πονηρῶν
πανδοχέων καὶ ἄλλων τινῶν.

—Galen, *De alimentorum facultatibus* III.1
(VI.661, 663K)

Pork

Pork is the most nourishing of all foods. Athletes provide the clearest proof of this. For if one day they replace their usual amount of pork with the same amount of a different food and pair that with their standard amount of exercise, on the next day they are already immediately weaker; if they keep doing this for multiple days in a row, they appear not just weaker but even visibly less well-nourished. . . . It is possible to know how similar pork is to human flesh from the fact that people have eaten human flesh passed off as pork without either the taste or the smell raising any suspicion (this has been revealed to be a practice of wicked innkeepers and the like).

—Galen, *On the Properties of Foodstuffs*

Perna:

Pernam, ubi eam cum caricis plurimis elixaveris et tribus lauri foliis, detracta cute tessellatim incidis et melle complebis. Deinde farinam oleo subactam contexes et ei coreum reddis ut, cum farina cocta fuerit, eximas furno et ut est inferes.

—*Apicius* VII.9.1

Beef

βοὸς κρέα ἰσχυρὰ καὶ στάσιμα καὶ δύσπεπτα τῇσι κοιλίῃσι, διότι παχύαιμον καὶ πουλύαιμόν ἐστι τὸ ζῶον.

—Hippocratic *De victu* II.46.1

τὰ δὲ βόεια κρέα τροφὴν μὲν καὶ αὐτὰ δίδωσιν οὔτ' ὀλίγην οὔτ' εὐδιαφόρητον, αἷμα

Recipe for ham:

When you have thoroughly boiled it with lots of dried figs and three bay leaves, take off its skin, score the ham in a checker pattern, and fill the cuts with honey. Then cover it in flour kneaded with oil and make this into a crust for it so that, once the flour is cooked, you can take it out of the oven and serve it as is.

—*Apicius' Cookbook*

Beef

Beef is strong and constipating and difficult for the bowels to digest because the animal has thick and abundant blood.

—Hippocratic *Regimen*

Beef also provides nourishment, but it is scant and difficult to incorporate and

μέντοι παχύτερον ἢ προσήκει γεννᾷ. καὶ εἰ
φύσει τις εἴη μελαγχολικώτερος τὴν κρᾶσιν, ἁλώσεταί τινι παθήματι τῶν μελαγχο-
λικῶν ἐν τῇ τούτων ἐδωδῇ πλεονάσας.
τοιαῦτα δ' ἐστὶ πάθη καρκίνος, ἐλέφας,
ψώρα, λέπρα, πυρετὸς τεταρταῖος ἤ τ'
ἰδίως ὀνομαζομένη μελαγχολία.

—Galen, *De alimentorum facultatibus* III.1
(VI.661–62K)

Other Meats

ὑγροτάτην δ' ἔχουσι καὶ φλεγματώδη
σάρκα καὶ οἱ ἄρνες. ἀλλὰ καὶ τῶν προβά-
των ἡ σὰρξ περιττωματικωτέρα τέ ἐστι καὶ
κακοχυμοτέρα. κακόχυμος δὲ καὶ ἡ τῶν
αἰγῶν μετὰ δριμύτητος. ἡ δὲ τῶν τράγων
χειρίστη καὶ πρὸς εὐχυμίαν καὶ πρὸς
πέψιν . . . καὶ τοῦ λαγωοῦ δ' ἡ σὰρξ αἵματος
μέν ἐστι παχυτέρου γεννητική, βελτίων
δ' εἰς εὐχυμίαν ἢ κατὰ βοῦς καὶ πρόβατα.

produces a thicker blood than is ideal. And anyone naturally of a rather melancholic constitution who overindulges in its consumption will be seized by one of the melancholic diseases. These diseases include: cancer, elephantiasis, psoriasis, scaly skin, quartan fever, and the one specifically called "melancholy."

—Galen, *On the Properties of Foodstuffs*

Other Meats

Lambs have an extremely moist and phlegm-producing flesh. But the flesh of grown sheep is more unwholesome and productive of residues. That of goats is unwholesome as well as pungent. That of he-goats is the worst, both in terms of wholesomeness and ease of digestion.... The flesh of hares is productive of a thick blood, but it is better in terms of wholesomeness than

κακόχυμος δὲ τούτων οὐδὲν ἧττόν ἐστι καὶ
ἡ τῶν ἐλάφων καὶ σκληρὰ καὶ δύσπεπτος. ἡ
δὲ τῶν ἀγρίων ὄνων, ὅσοι γ' εὔεκται καὶ
νέοι, πλησίον ἥκει τῆσδε. καίτοι καὶ τῶν
ἡμέρων ὄνων γηρασάντων ἔνιοι τὰ κρέα
προσφέρονται, κακοχυμότατά τε καὶ δυσ-
πεπτότατα καὶ κακοστόμαχα καὶ προσέτι
καὶ ἀηδῆ κατὰ τὴν ἐδωδὴν ὄντα, καθάπερ
καὶ τὰ τῶν ἵππων τε καὶ καμήλων, ὧν καὶ
αὐτῶν ἐσθίουσιν οἱ ὀνώδεις τε καὶ καμηλώ-
δεις ἄνθρωποι τήν τε ψυχὴν καὶ τὸ σῶμα.

—Galen, *De alimentorum facultatibus* III.1
(VI.663–64K)

Poultry

ὁ δὲ ζωμὸς τοῦ νόσσακος μάλιστα δίδοται
ἐπικράσεως χάριν φαυλοτήτων.

—Dioscorides, *De materia medica* II.49

beef or mutton. Venison is no less unwholesome than those are, being both tough and indigestible. The flesh of the wild ass (those that are young and in good shape) is almost as good as venison; however, some people also serve meat from old, domesticated donkeys, which is extremely unwholesome, extremely difficult to digest, and bad for the stomach, besides being distasteful to eat, just like the flesh of horses and camels (people who eat them are asinine and camel-like, body and soul).

— Galen, *On the Properties of Foodstuffs*

Poultry

Chicken soup is very often given to those in poor health in order to set them to rights.

— Dioscorides, *Medical Substances*

ὀρνίθων . . . σχεδόν τι πάντα ξηρότερα ἢ τὰ
τετράποδα. ὅσα γὰρ κύστιν οὐκ ἔχει, οὔτε
οὐρεῖ οὔτε σιαλοχοεῖ διὰ θερμότητα τῆς
κοιλίης· . . . ξηρότατον μὲν οὖν φαίνεται
φάσσης, δεύτερον πέρδικος, τρίτον περι-
στερῆς καὶ ἀλεκτρυόνος καὶ τρυγόνος·
ὑγρότατον δὲ χηνός. ὅσα δὲ σπερμολογεῖ
ξηρότερα τῶν ἑτέρων. νήσσης δὲ καὶ τῶν
ἄλλων, ὅσα ἐν ἕλεσι διαιτᾶται ἢ ἐν ὕδατι,
πάντα ὑγρά.

—Hippocratic *De victu* II.47.1–2

Eggs

τῆς ἀπὸ τῶν πτηνῶν ζῴων τροφῆς ἐστι καὶ
ταῦτα διαφέροντα τρισὶ διαφοραῖς ἀλλήλων, μιᾷ μὲν τῇ κατὰ τὴν οἰκείαν οὐσίαν
(ἀμείνω γὰρ τά τε τῶν ἀλεκτορίδων ἐστὶ
καὶ τὰ τῶν φασιανῶν, φαυλότερα δὲ τὰ τῶν
χηνῶν τε καὶ στρουθοκαμήλων), ἑτέρᾳ δέ,

Just about all birds are drier than four-footed animals (for anything that does not have a bladder neither urinates nor salivates on account of the heat of its belly). . . . The driest flesh seems to be that of the ring-dove, in second place the partridge, in third the pigeon, the rooster, and the turtle-dove; the moistest is the goose. Those that eat seeds are drier than the others. The duck and the other types that spend their time in marshland or in water are all moist.

—Hippocratic *Regimen*

Eggs

These are also a type of nourishment derived from poultry, and they differ from each other in three respects: in the first place, according to their natural type (chicken and pheasant eggs are better, goose and ostrich worse); second, according to

καθ' ἣν τὰ μὲν ἤδη χρόνου πλείονός ἐστι,
τὰ δ' οὐ πρὸ πολλοῦ γεγέννηται, καὶ τρίτῃ,
καθ' ἣν τὰ μὲν ἐπὶ πλέον ἥψηται, τὰ δ' ἄχρι
τοῦ μετρίως συστῆναι, τὰ δὲ μόνον τεθέρ-
μανται· καθ' ἃς διαφορὰς τὰ μὲν ἑφθὰ καλεῖται, τὰ δὲ τρομητά, τὰ δὲ ῥοφητά.

κάλλιστα μὲν οὖν αὐτῶν ἐστιν εἰς τροφὴν
τοῦ σώματος τὰ τρομητά, τὰ ῥοφητὰ δ'
ἧττον μὲν τρέφει, ῥᾷον δ' ὑποχωρεῖ καὶ τὰς
ἐν τῇ φάρυγγι τραχύτητας ἐκλεαίνει. τὰ δ'
ἑφθὰ καὶ δύσπεπτα καὶ βραδύπορα, καὶ
τροφὴν παχεῖαν ἀναδίδωσι τῷ σώματι. τούτων δ' ἔτι μᾶλλόν ἐστι βραδυπορώτερά τε
καὶ παχυχυμότερα τὰ κατὰ θερμὴν σποδιὰν
ὀπτηθέντα. τὰ δ' ἐπὶ τῶν ταγήνων παχυν-
θέντα καὶ καλούμενα διὰ τοῦτο ταγηνιστὰ
χειρίστην ἔχει τροφὴν εἰς ἅπαντα· καὶ γὰρ ἐν
τῷ πέττεσθαι κνισοῦται καὶ πρὸς τῷ παχὺν
γεννᾶν χυμὸν ἔτι καὶ μοχθηρὸν ἔχει καὶ
περιττωματικὸν αὐτόν. . . .

their age (some sit around for a long time, others were only just laid); third, according to their preparation (some were boiled for a while, others just until they got moderately firm, others were only warmed—the first in this category are called hard-boiled, the second soft-boiled, the third runny).

Soft-boiled eggs are the best of these in terms of nourishment for the body; runny ones nourish less but go down easily and smooth away roughness in the throat. Hard-boiled eggs are both difficult to digest and difficult to pass, and they provide a thick nutriment to the body. Even harder to pass and thicker than these are the ones cooked on hot ashes. But the ones set on a frying pan (and for this reason called fried) have the worst nutriment in all respects: for in the cooking process they become greasy and, in addition to producing a thick humor, they also contain a pernicious one, full of residues. . . .

οὐ σμικρὰ δ' ἐν αὐτοῖς ἐστιν ὑπεροχὴ καὶ τῶν νέων πρὸς τὰ παλαιά· κάλλιστα μὲν γὰρ τὰ νεώτατα, χείριστα δὲ τὰ παλαιότατα, τὰ δ' ἐν τῷ μεταξὺ τούτων ἀνὰ λόγον τῆς ἀποστάσεως, ἧς ἀφέστηκε τῶν ἄκρων, ἀρετῇ τε καὶ κακίᾳ διενήνοχεν ἀλλήλων.

—Galen, *De alimentorum facultatibus* III.21 (VI.705–7K)

The degree of superiority among eggs is also not inconsiderable when it comes to new ones over old ones. For the newest ones are the best, the oldest ones are the worst, and the ones between these differ among themselves with respect to goodness and badness in proportion to the degree to which they are distant from the extremes.

—Galen, *On the Properties of Foodstuffs*

Fish

ἥ γε μὴν τροφὴ κἀκ τοῦδε κἀκ τῶν ἄλλων
ἰχθύων αἵματός ἐστι γεννητικὴ λεπτοτέρου
τῇ συστάσει τῆς ἐκ τῶν πεζῶν ζῴων, ὡς
μήτε τρέφειν δαψιλῶς καὶ διαφορεῖσθαι

FISH AND SEAFOOD

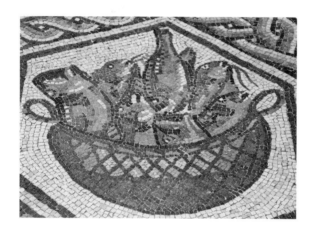

Fish

The nourishment from sea bass and from
other fish is productive of a blood thinner
in composition than that derived from
eating land animals, so it does not nourish

θᾶττον. . . . ἄριστον δὲ τὸ τούτων ἀκριβῶς
μεταξὺ γεννώμενον ἐξ ἄρτου τε τοῦ κάλλιστα κατεσκευασμένου . . . καὶ τῶν πτηνῶν
ὧν εἴρηται ζῴων, ἐκ πέρδικός τε καὶ τῶν
παραπλησίων. ἐγγὺς δὲ τούτων εἰσὶ καὶ τῶν
θαλαττίων οἱ πελάγιοι τῶν ἰχθύων. . . .
ἁπάντων δὲ τῶν εἰρημένων ἰχθύων ἡ τροφὴ
καλλίστη τοῖς τε μὴ γυμναζομένοις ἐστὶ καὶ
ἀργοῦσι καὶ ἀσθενέσι καὶ τοῖς ἐκνοσηλευο-
μένοις· οἱ γυμναζόμενοι δὲ τροφιμωτέρων
ἐδεσμάτων δέονται, περὶ ὧν ἔμπροσθεν
εἴρηται.

—Galen, *De alimentorum facultatibus*
III.25, 29 (VI.714–15, 726K)

ἐπὶ πάντων δ', ὡς ἔφην, ἰχθύων κοινὸν
τοῦτο μεμνῆσθαι προσήκει, ὡς χείριστοι γί-
γνονται κατὰ τὰς ἐκβολὰς τῶν ποταμῶν,

abundantly and is quickly dissipated. . . .
The best blood—the one produced exactly between the two extremes of thick
and thin—comes from bread that has been
prepared in the best possible way . . . and
from the partridge and birds similar to it
(of the winged animals that I mentioned).
But deep-sea saltwater fish come close to
these. . . . The nourishment from all the
types of fish mentioned here is most suitable for people who are not exercising but
who are idle and feeble and convalescing.
Those who exercise require more nourishing foods, as I have said before.

—Galen, *On the Properties of Foodstuffs*

It is a good idea, as I mentioned, to remember this fact common to all fish: they
are of the worst quality when found at the

ὅσοι κοπρῶνας ἐκκαθαίρουσιν ἢ βαλανεῖα
καὶ μαγειρεῖα καὶ τὸν τῆς ἐσθῆτός τε καὶ τὸν
τῶν ὀθονίων ῥύπον ὅσα τ' ἄλλα τῆς πόλεώς
ἐστιν, ἣν διαρρέουσι, καθάρσεως δεόμενα,
καὶ μάλισθ' ὅταν ᾖ πολυάνθρωπος ἡ πόλις.

—Galen, *De alimentorum facultatibus* III.29
(VI.721–22K)

Thynni . . . membratim caesi cervice et
abdomine commendantur atque clidio,
recenti dumtaxat, et tum quoque gravi
ructu; cetera parte plenis pulpamentis sale
adservantur: melandrya vocantur, quercus
assulis similia. Vilissima ex his quae caudae
proxima, quia pingui carent, probatissima
quae faucibus; at in alio pisce circa caudam
exercitatissima. . . .

mouths of any river that clears out latrines or bathhouses or cookshops or the waste-water from clothes and linens and anything else requiring washing in the city through which it runs (especially if the city is very populous).

—Galen, *On the Properties of Foodstuffs*

Tuna, cut up into pieces, are valued for their neck, abdomen, and collar bone, at least while they are fresh (even though they cause heavy belching). The rest of the tuna is preserved in parts in salt, with all the meat intact: these are called "oak-hearts" and look similar to shingles of oak. The worst of these are the parts closest to the tail, because they lack fat; the most prized are the ones closest to the jaws (though in other fish, the part near the tail is the most frequently used). . . .

Nunc principatus scaro datur, qui solus piscium dicitur ruminare herbisque vesci atque non aliis piscibus. . . . Ex reliqua nobilitate et gratia maxima est et copia mullis, sicut magnitudo modica, binasque libras ponderis raro admodum exuperant, nec in vivariis piscinisque crescunt. . . . M. Apicius ad omne luxus ingenium natus in sociorum garo—nam ea quoque res cognomen invenit—necari eos praecellens putavit, atque e iecore eorum alecem excogitari. . . .

Est et haec natura ut alii alibi pisces principatum optineant, coracinus in Aegypto, zaeus, idem faber appellatus, Gadibus, circa Ebusum salpa. Obscenus alibi et qui nusquam percoqui possit nisi ferula verberatus;

At the present time, the first rank of popularity is given to the parrotfish, which are said to be the only fish that ruminate like a cow and eat plants rather than other fish. . . . Of the other popular fish, the highest spot for both pleasure and abundance goes to the mullets, even though they are modest in size (they very rarely exceed two pounds in weight and don't even grow larger in aquariums and pools). . . . Marcus Apicius (a man born with a genius for all kinds of luxury) thinks it an excellent thing for them to be killed in a sauce made of their companion fish (this, too, has found a name for itself: garum) and for fish-paste to be made from their livers. . . .

And it is natural, too, that different fish occupy the first rank of popularity in different places: the raven fish in Egypt, the *zaeus* (also called the dory) in Cadiz, the cow bream in the areas around Ibiza

in Aquitania salmo fluviatilis marinis omnibus praefertur.

—Pliny the Elder, *Naturalis historia* IX.18.48, 29.62, 30.64, 32.68

Mollusks and Crustaceans

κοινὸν μὲν οὖν ἁπάντων τῶν τοιούτων ἁλυκὸν ἔχειν χυμὸν ἐν τῇ σαρκὶ λαπακτικὸν τῆς γαστρὸς ἡμῶν. ἴδιον δ᾽ ἑκάστῳ τὸ μᾶλλόν τε καὶ ἧττον ἐν τούτῳ κατά τε ποιότητα καὶ ποσότητα. τὰ μὲν γὰρ ὄστρεα μαλακωτάτην ἔχει τῶν ἄλλων ὀστρακοδέρμων ἁπάντων τὴν σάρκα, τὰ δὲ σμικρὰ χημία καὶ οἱ σωλῆνες καὶ οἱ σφόνδυλοι καὶ αἱ πορφύραι καὶ οἱ κήρυκες ὅσα τ᾽ ἄλλα τοιαῦτα σκληράν. εἰκότως οὖν ὑπάγει μὲν ἐκεῖνα τὴν γαστέρα μᾶλλον, ἥττονα τροφὴν διδόντα τῷ σώματι· τὰ δὲ σκληρόσαρκα δυσπεπτότερα μέν ἐστι, τρέφει δὲ μᾶλλον. ἀλλὰ ταῦτα μὲν

(though it is disgusting elsewhere and unable to be cooked unless first beaten with a stick); in Aquitaine, the river salmon is preferred to all marine fish.

—Pliny the Elder, *Natural History*

Mollusks and Crustaceans

A common element to all these sorts of animals is the possession of a salty juice in their flesh that is laxative to our bellies. This exists to a greater or lesser degree in each animal, both in terms of its quality and its quantity. Oysters have the softest flesh of all the mollusks, but small clams, razor clams, spiny oysters, murex snails, trumpet snails, and others like these have hard flesh. So it is reasonable that oysters empty the stomach more, while providing less nourishment to the body; but the hard-fleshed ones are more difficult to digest,

ἕψεται πάντα, τὰ δ' ὄστρεα χωρὶς ἑψήσεως
ἐσθίουσιν, ἔνιοι δὲ καὶ ταγηνίζουσιν. . . .

ἀστακοὶ καὶ πάγουροι καρκίνοι τε καὶ κά-
ραβοι καὶ καρῖδες καὶ καμμαρίδες ὅσα τ'
ἄλλα λεπτὸν μὲν ἔχει τὸ περιέχον ὄστρακον,
ὅμοιον δὲ τῇ σκληρότητι τοῖς ὀστρακο-
δέρμοις, ἥττονα μὲν ἐκείνων ἔχει τὸν ἁλυκὸν χυμόν, ἔχει δ' οὖν ὅμως οὐκ ὀλίγον.
ἐστὶ δὲ σκληρόσαρκα πάντα καὶ διὰ τοῦτο
δύσπεπτά τε καὶ τρόφιμα, προεψηθέντα
δηλονότι κατὰ τὸ πότιμον ὕδωρ.

—Galen, *De alimentorum facultatibus*
III.32–33 (VI.734–36K)

Iam quidem ex tota rerum natura damno-
sissimum ventri mare est tot modis, tot

but more nourishing. But, whereas all these latter are boiled, people eat oysters without cooking them (though some people do fry them). . . .

Lobsters, brown crabs, rock crabs, crayfish, shrimp, spiny lobsters, and any others that have a surrounding shell that is thin, but similar to that of mollusks in terms of hardness: these have less salty humor than mollusks do, but it is still not inconsiderable. They are all hard-fleshed and, for this reason, difficult to digest but nourishing (obviously, having first been boiled in potable water).

—Galen, *On the Properties of Foodstuffs*

Of the whole of the natural world, the sea is the most destructive to the stomach, with so many varieties, so many dishes, so many flavors of seafood, whose

mensis, tot piscium saporibus quis pretia capientium periculo fiunt.

—Pliny the Elder, *Naturalis historia* IX.53.104–5

Quid? Illa ostrea, inertissimam carnem caeno saginatam, nihil existimas limosae gravitatis inferre?

—Seneca, *Epistulae* 95.25

high value tempts those who catch them into danger.

—Pliny the Elder, *Natural History*

What? Do you really think that oysters— the world's most sluggish flesh, fattened on mud—bring no slimy heaviness to the body?

—Seneca, *Letters*

COMPOUND DISHES

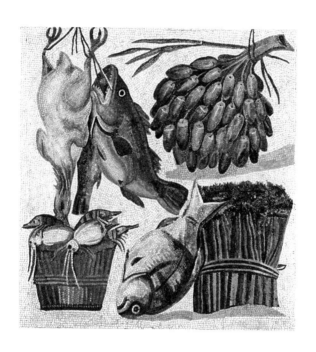

ὠφελείας γὰρ ἡμεῖς στοχαζόμεθα τῆς ἐκ
τῶν ἐδεσμάτων, οὐχ ἡδονῆς. ἐπεὶ δ᾽ ἐνίων
ἡ κατὰ τὴν ἐδωδὴν ἀηδία μέγα μέρος εἰς
ἀπεψίαν συμβάλλεται, κατὰ τοῦτο μετρίως
ἡδύνειν αὐτὰ βέλτιόν ἐστιν. ἡ δὲ τῶν μαγεί-
ρων ἡδονὴ μοχθηροῖς οὕτως ἀρτύμασιν ὡς
τὸ πολὺ χρῆται συνήθως, ὡς ἀπεψίαν μᾶλλον ἢ εὐπεψίαν αὐτοῖς ἕπεσθαι.

—Galen, *De alimentorum facultatibus* II.51
(VI.639K)

Nec est mirum tunc illam minus negotii
habuisse firmis adhuc solidisque corporibus
et facili cibo nec per artem voluptatemque
corrupto: qui postquam coepit non ad tol-
lendam sed ad inritandam famem quaeri et
inventae sunt mille conditurae quibus avi-
ditas excitaretur, quae desiderantibus alim-
enta erant onera sunt plenis. . . . Simplex erat
ex causa simplici valetudo: multos morbos

We doctors aim to achieve benefit from the things people eat, not pleasure. Of course, since distaste for the things you eat is sometimes in large part responsible for poor digestion, it is better for things to be reasonably appealing. But, for cooks, pleasurable taste is usually obtained by seasonings that are so pernicious that they actually lead to poor digestion rather than improving it.

— Galen, *On the Properties of Foodstuffs*

It is not surprising that the field of medicine used to have less business: people used to have sound and solid bodies and eat simple food that was not corrupted by the art of pleasure. Since then, people have begun to hunt for ways to rouse hunger, rather than to satisfy it, and thousands of dishes have been invented by which to excite an appetite. We used to have food for

multa fericula fecerunt. Vide quantum rerum per unam gulam transiturarum permisceat luxuria, terrarum marisque vastatrix. Nec-esse est itaque inter se tam diversa dissi-deant et hausta male digerantur aliis alio nitentibus. Nec mirum quod inconstans variusque ex discordi cibo morbus est et illa ex contrariis naturae partibus in eundem conpulsa <ventrem> redundant. . . . Innum-erabiles esse morbos non miraberis: cocos numera. . . .

Memini fuisse quondam in sermone nobilem patinam in quam quidquid apud lautos solet diem ducere properans in damnum suum popina congesserat: veneriae

hungry stomachs; now we have burdens for full ones. . . . Simple heath came from simple causes: a wild multiplicity of choices yields a multiplicity of diseases. Consider how many things luxurious living will mix together to be stuffed down a single throat: it ravages the land and sea. It is inevitable that such a diversity of foods will disagree with each other, and once swallowed they are digested badly, each struggling against the others. Nor is it surprising that the diseases arising from discordant food are various and changeable and that something has to give when things with contrary natures are stuffed into the same stomach. . . . Don't be shocked that there are countless diseases: count the cooks instead. . . .

I recall once hearing tell of a celebrated casserole, in which a cookshop (hastening itself toward financial ruin) mixed together whatever was in fad with the elegant:

spondylique et ostrea eatenus circumcisa qua
eduntur intervenientibus distinguebantur
†echini totam destructique† sine ullis ossibus
mulli constraverant. Piget esse iam singula:
coguntur in unum sapores. In cena fit quod
fieri debebat in ventre: expecto iam ut
manducata ponantur. . . . Non esset confu-
sior vomentium cibus. Quomodo ista per-
plexa sunt, sic ex istis non singulares morbi
nascuntur sed inexplicabiles, diversi, multi-
formes, adversus quos et medicina armare
se coepit multis generibus, multis obser-
vationibus.

—Seneca, *Epistulae* 95.15, 18–19, 23, 26–29

cockles and mussels and oysters (the edible part only, having been cut out of the shells), interlaced with whole sea urchins and surrounded by deboned fillets of mullet. These days, one food at a time is disgusting: people like lots of flavors in one dish. What is supposed to happen in your stomach now happens on your dinner plate: it's just a matter of time before things are served prechewed. . . . Vomited food could not be more mixed up. So how is it perplexing that not just a few diseases have arisen from them, but diverse, multifaceted, and intransigent ones, against which the art of medicine is only beginning to arm itself through much trial and observation.

—Seneca, *Letters*

Patinam ex lacte:

Nucleos infundes et siccas; echinos recentes iam praeparatos habebis. Accipies patinam et in eam compones singula infra scriptam:

mediana maluarum et betarum et porros
    maturos
apios holus molles et viridia elixa
pullum carptum ex iure coctum
cerebella elixa
lucania
ova dura per medium incisa

Mittes:

longaones porcinos ex iure Terentino
    farsos coctos concisos
iecinera pullorum
pulpas piscis ascelli fricti
urticas marinas
pulpas hostreorum
caseos recentes

Recipe for a Casserole with Milk:

Soak some pine nuts and put them to dry. You should have some fresh sea urchins already prepared. Take a casserole dish and put in any of the ingredients listed below:

tender insides of mallow plants and
    beetroots and some full-grown leeks
parsley, gentle herbs, and boiled greens
bits of chicken meat, cooked in broth
boiled brains
smoked sausages
hard-boiled eggs, cut in half

Add:

pork sausages, stuffed with Terentine
    sauce, cooked, and cut into pieces
chicken livers
flaked haddock
sea-nettles
oyster meat
freshly made cheese

Alternis conpones nucleos et piper integrum asparges. Ius tale perfundes:

    piper
    ligusticum
    apii semen
    silfi

Quoques, at ubi cocta fuerit lactem colas cui cruda ova conmisces ut unum corpus fiat et super illa omnia perfundes. Cum cocta fuerit <conpones> echinos recentiores, piper asparges et inferes.

—*Apicius* IV.2.13

Place them together in alternating layers, and sprinkle with the pine nuts and whole pepper. Pour in a sauce made like this:

pepper
lovage
celery seed
silphium[1]

Cook. When it is cooked, whisk milk to which you have added raw egg until it is uniform in texture and pour it in over everything. When that is cooked, put on your fresh sea urchins, sprinkle on some pepper, and serve.

—*Apicius' Cookbook*

Figs

τροφὴν δ᾽ ἁπασῶν τῶν ὀπωρῶν ὀλίγην τῷ
σώματι διδουσῶν, ἧττον ἁπασῶν τοῦτο τὰ
σῦκα πέπονθεν, οὐ μὴν ἐσφιγμένην γε
καὶ ἰσχυρὰν ἐργάζεται τὴν σάρκα, καθάπερ

FRUITS, NUTS, AND SWEETS

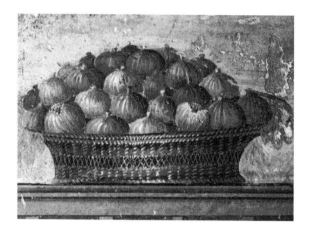

Figs

Although it is the case that all fruits give little nourishment to the body, figs are the least problematic in this regard, though they certainly do not produce a firm and

ἄρτος τε καὶ κρέας ὕειον, ἀλλ᾽ ὑπόσομφον
ὥσπερ ὁ κύαμος. ἐμπίπλησί γε μὴν φύσης
καὶ αὐτὰ τὴν γαστέρα, καὶ ἦν ἂν ἱκανῶς
ταύτῃ λυπηρά, μὴ προσλαβόντα τὸ διαχω-
ρεῖσθαι ταχέως, ἐπικτησάμενα δὲ τοῦτο τῷ
τάχει τῆς διεξόδου τὴν φῦσαν ὀλιγοχρόνιον
ἐργάζεται, καὶ κατὰ τοῦτ᾽ αὐτὸ τῆς ἄλλης
ὀπώρας ἧττον εἴωθε βλάπτειν. . . . τὸ γάρ
τοι πέπειρον ἀκριβῶς σῦκον ἐγγὺς τοῦ μηδ᾽
ὅλως βλάπτειν ἥκει, παραπλήσιον ἤδη ταῖς
ἰσχάσι, πολλὰ μὲν ἐχούσαις τὰ χρήσιμα, μοχθηρὸν δ᾽ ἕν τι τοῖς πλεονάζουσιν ἐν αὐταῖς.
οὐ πάνυ γὰρ αἷμα γεννῶσι χρηστόν, ὅθεν
αὐταῖς καὶ τὸ τῶν φθειρῶν πλῆθος ἕπεται.

—Galen, *De alimentorum facultatibus* II.8
(VI.571–72K)

strong flesh, like bread and pork do, but a somewhat flabby one, like beans produce. Indeed, even figs fill the stomach with air, and they would be quite troublesome in this regard except that they are also inclined to pass through quickly; due to this extra property, they cause only short-lived gas because of the speed of their passage and, as a result, they seem to be less harmful than any other fruit. . . . In fact, a perfectly ripened fig comes close to being entirely harmless, just like the dried ones. The dried ones are extremely useful, though they do have one pernicious quality for people who overindulge in them: they produce a blood that is not fully useable, from which follows an abundance of head lice.[1]

—Galen, *On the Properties of Foodstuffs*

οὗτος οὖν με παῖδα μὲν ὄντα διαιτῶν αὐτὸς
ἄνοσον ἐφύλαξεν. ἐπεὶ δὲ μειράκιον ἐγενό-
μην ὅ τε πατὴρ ὑπεχώρησεν εἰς ἀγρὸν ὢν
φιλογέωργος, εἰχόμην μὲν ὧν ἐμάνθανον
ὑπὲρ ἅπαντας τοὺς συμφοιτῶντας, οὐ δι᾽
ἡμέρας μόνον ἀλλὰ καὶ νύκτωρ. ἐμπλησθεὶς
δὲ μετὰ τῶν ἡλικιωτῶν ἐν ἅπαντι τῷ χρόνῳ
τῆς ὀπώρας ἁπάντων τῶν ὡραίων ἐνόσησα
τοῦ φθινοπώρου νόσον ὀξεῖαν, ὡς φλεβο-
τομίας δεηθῆναι. παραγενόμενος οὖν εἰς
τὴν πόλιν ὁ πατὴρ ἐπετίμησέ τέ μοι καὶ τῆς
ἔμπροσθεν ἀνέμνησε διαίτης, ἣν ὑπ᾽ αὐτῷ
διῃτώμην, ἐκέλευσέ τε τοῦ λοιποῦ φυλάτ-
τειν αὐτὴν ἀποστάντα τῆς τῶν ἡλικιωτῶν
ἀκρασίας.... τῶν ὡραίων ἁπάντων ἐπέχειν ἐμαυτὸν ὥρισα πλὴν τῶν πεπείρων
ἀκριβῶς σύκων τε καὶ σταφυλῶν, οὐδὲ
τούτων ἀμέτρως, ὡς ἔμπροσθεν, ἀλλὰ συμμέτρως προσφερόμενος.

—Galen, *De bonis malisque sucis* 1.15–17, 19
(VI.755–57K)

When I was a child, my father himself took charge of keeping me on a healthy diet, but when I was a teenager, he withdrew to our country estate, being fond of farming. Although I was more obedient, both day and night, to the lifestyle I had been taught than any of my friends were, I nevertheless followed their example in gorging myself constantly on all the fruits in season, and in the autumn I fell ill with an acute disease, requiring bloodletting. My father, returning to the city, upbraided me and reminded me of my former diet, which I had observed under his guidance, and ordered me to follow it from then on and foreswear the intemperance of my contemporaries. . . . I made it a rule for myself to avoid all fruits except for perfectly ripened figs and grapes—and to not employ those immoderately as before, but in moderate amounts.

—Galen, *On Good and Bad Juices*

Apples

ἔνια μὲν γὰρ αὐστηρὸν ἔχει χυμόν, ἔνια δ᾽
ὀξὺν ἢ γλυκύν, ἔστι δ᾽ ἃ καὶ μικτὸν ἐκ τούτων, ὡς ἅμα τε γλυκέα φαίνεσθαι καὶ στύφοντα, καί τινα ἕτερα μετὰ γλυκύτητος
ὀξέα σαφῶς φαίνεται καὶ πρὸς τούτοις
ἄλλα στρυφνὰ μετ᾽ ὀξύτητος. . . . φυλάττεσθαι δὲ χρὴ καὶ τὰ κάλλιστα τῷ γένει μῆλα
πρὶν ἐπὶ τῶν δένδρων πεπανθῆναι. δύσπεπτά τε γάρ ἐστι καὶ βραδυπόρα καὶ κακόχυμα μετὰ τοῦ καὶ ψυχρὸν καὶ παχὺν ἀτρέμα
τὸν χυμὸν ἔχειν. ὅσα δὲ καλῶς πεπανθέντα
φυλάττουσιν εἴς τε τὸν χειμῶνα καὶ τὸ μετ᾽
αὐτὸν ἔαρ, ὠφελιμώτατα γίγνεται πολλάκις ἐν νόσοις, ἤτοι περιπλασθέντα σταιτὶ
καὶ κατὰ θερμὴν σποδιὰν ὀπτηθέντα συμμέτρως ἢ ἐν ὕδατος ζέοντος ἀτμῷ καλῶς
ἑψηθέντα.

—Galen, *De alimentorum facultatibus* II.21
(VI.594, 597K)

Apples

Some apples have a bitter juice, others sharp or sweet, and there are even some that have a mixture of these flavors, so that they appear simultaneously sweet and tart, and in some others a sharpness is clearly discernable alongside their sweetness while others are tart alongside their sharpness. . . . It is necessary to be wary of even the best kind of apples before they have ripened on the tree. For they are difficult to digest, slow to pass through, and unwholesome, with a juice that is both cold and slightly thick. But those that were well-ripened and stored away for the winter and the following spring are often extremely useful in illnesses, if they are wrapped in pastry and evenly baked over hot ashes or else well stewed in the steam of boiling water.

—Galen, *On the Properties of Foodstuffs*

Poma nocere quidam putant, quae inmodice toto die plerumque sic adsumuntur, ne quid ex densiore cibo remittatur. Ita non haec sed consummatio omnium nocet; ex quibus in nullo tamen minus quam in his noxae est. Sed his uti non saepius quam alio cibo convenit. Denique aliquid densiori cibo, cum hic accedit, necessarium est demi.

—Celsus, *De medicina* I.3

Peaches

Pomum innocuum expetitur aegris, pretiumque iam singulis triceni nummi fuere, nullius maiore, quod miremur, quia non aliud fugacius: longissima namque

Some people think that apples are harmful; they certainly are if you go overboard and eat them all day long and don't cut back on one of the denser foods. In this case, it's not the apples themselves, but the way you have approached your diet as whole, that is harmful. In fact, no part of your diet is less harmful than them. But you should eat them no more frequently than any other food; and, when you add them to your diet, be sure to cut back on one of the denser foods.

—Celsus, *On Medicine*

Peaches

This harmless fruit is sought after by the ailing, and a single one has gone for a price of thirty sesterces, more than any other fruit—which is astonishing because no other fruit keeps worse. The longest it lasts

decerpto bidui mora est cogitque se ven-
umdari.

—Pliny the Elder, *Naturalis historia* XV.11.40

ἤδη δ᾽ ἴσθι . . . ὡς καὶ τούτων ὁ χυλός τε καὶ
ἡ οἷον σὰρξ εὔφθαρτός τ᾽ ἐστι καὶ πάντη
μοχθηρά. ὥστ᾽ οὐ χρή, καθάπερ ἔνιοι, τελευταῖα τῆς ἄλλης τροφῆς αὐτὰ προσφέ-
ρεσθαι· διαφθείρεται γὰρ ἐπιπολάζοντα.
μεμνῆσθαι δὲ χρὴ τοῦδε κοινοῦ πάντων
ὄντος, ὡς τὰ κακόχυμα μέν, ὑγρὰ δὲ καὶ
ὀλισθηρὰ καὶ ῥᾳδίως ὑπιέναι δυνάμενα διὰ
τοῦτ᾽ ἐσθίειν δεῖ πρότερα τῶν ἄλλων· οὕτω
γὰρ αὐτά τε ταχέως ὑπέρχεται κἀκείνοις
ποδηγεῖ· τὰ δ᾽ ὕστατα ληφθέντα συνδια-
φθείρει καὶ τἄλλα.

—Galen, *De alimentorum facultatibus* II.19
(VI.592–93K)

after picking is two days: it begs to be sold.

—Pliny the Elder, *Natural History*

Indeed, you should know . . . that the juice and the fleshly part of these fruits, too, is easily corrupted and completely pernicious. So that you should not—like some do—take these as a final course after the rest of the meal; for they linger in the stomach and decompose. Remember this common rule for all foods: things that are unwholesome and things that are moist, slippery, and easily slide down ought, for this reason, to be eaten before other foods: for they descend quickly, as is their nature, and serve as a guide for the rest. But taken at the end, they decompose everything else along with themselves.

—Galen, *On the Properties of Foodstuffs*

Nuts

πολλὴ δ᾽ ἀμφοτέρων ἡ χρῆσίς ἐστιν οὐ πολλὴν τροφὴν διδόντων τῷ σώματι . . . πέττεταί γε μὴν μᾶλλον τὸ κάρυον τοῦ λεπτοκαρύου καὶ μᾶλλον εὐστόμαχόν ἐστι, καὶ πολὺ μᾶλλον ὅταν σὺν ἰσχάσιν ἐσθίηται. γέγραπται δ᾽ ὑπὸ πολλῶν ἰατρῶν, ὡς ἐὰν ἄμφω ταῦτα πρὸ τῶν ἄλλων σιτίων λαμβάνηται μετὰ πηγάνου, μηδὲν ὑπὸ τῶν θανασίμων φαρμάκων μέγα βλαβήσεσθαι τὸν ἄνθρωπον. . . . <πιστάκια> τροφὴν μὲν ὀλιγίστην ἔχοντα, χρήσιμα δ᾽ εἰς ἥπατος εὐρωστίαν . . .

—Galen, *De alimentorum facultatibus* II.28, 30 (VI.609–10, 612K)

Nuces abellanae capitis dolorem faciunt et inflationem stomachi, corpori etiam pinguitudinis conferunt plus quam sit verisimile. . . . pistacia eosdem usus habent

Nuts

Much use is made of both varieties of walnuts even though they do not give much nourishment to the body. . . . The "royal" walnut is more easily digested than the thin-shelled variety and easier on the stomach, especially if it is eaten with dried figs. Many doctors are on record that if a person eats either variety, together with rue, before other foods, then poisonous drugs will do them no great harm. . . . Pistachios offer little nourishment, but are useful for strengthening the liver.

—Galen, *On the Properties of Foodstuffs*

Hazelnuts cause headaches and bloating in the stomach; further, they cause the body to put on more fat than seems credible. . . . Pistachios are used in the same way as pine

quos nuclei pinei praeterque ad serpentium ictus, sive edantur sive bibantur. Castaneae vehementer sistunt stomachi et ventris fluctiones, alvum cient, sanguinem excreantibus prosunt, carnes alunt.

—Pliny the Elder, *Naturalis historia* XXIII.78.150

Honey

ἔναγχος γοῦν ἐφιλονείκουν ἀλλήλοις δύο τινές, ὁ μὲν ὑγιεινὸν ἀποφαινόμενος, ὁ δὲ νοσερὸν εἶναι τὸ μέλι, τεκμαιρόμενος ἑκάτερος ἐξ ὧν αὐτὸς ὑπ' αὐτοῦ διετίθετο, μηκέτ' ἐννοοῦντες, ὡς οὔτε μίαν ἅπαντες ἄνθρωποι τὴν ἐξ ἀρχῆς ἔχουσι κρᾶσιν οὔτ', εἰ καὶ μίαν εἶχον, ἀμετάβλητον αὐτὴν ἐν ταῖς ἡλικίαις φυλάττουσιν, ὥσπερ οὐδ' ἐν ταῖς κατὰ τὰς ὥρας τε καὶ χώρας ὑπαλλαγαῖς, ἵνα παραλίπω κατά γε τὸ παρόν, ὡς καὶ τοῖς

nuts and, in addition, are effective against snake bites, whether eaten or drunk. Chestnuts bring fluxes in both stomach and belly firmly to a standstill, encourage good bowel movement, benefit those who cough up blood, and nourish the flesh.

—Pliny the Elder, *Natural History*

Honey

Recently, two people were quarreling with each other, one of them declaring that honey is healthy, the other that it is unhealthy, each one giving evidence from his own experiences of it, neither one of them being aware that all people do not have a single constitution from birth nor, even if they did all have a single one, would they keep it unaltered as they aged (and similarly not as they changed seasons or locales—and I won't even digress into how

ἐπιτηδεύμασι καὶ ταῖς διαίταις ὑπαλλάτ-
τουσι τὰς φυσικὰς τῶν σωμάτων διαθέ-
σεις. εὐθὺς γοῦν αὐτῶν τῶν διαφερομένων
ἀλλήλοις περὶ τοῦ μέλιτος ὁ μὲν πρεσβύτης
τε κατὰ τὴν ἡλικίαν ἦν καὶ φύσει φλεγματω-
δέστερος ἀργός τε τῷ βίῳ καὶ πρὸς τὰς
ἄλλας μὲν ἁπάσας πράξεις, οὐχ ἥκιστα δὲ
καὶ τὰ πρὸ τοῦ βαλανείου γυμνάσια, καὶ διὰ
τοῦτ᾽ αὐτῷ τὸ μέλι χρήσιμον ἦν· ὁ δ᾽ ἕτερος
χολώδης τε φύσει καὶ τριακοντούτης κατὰ
τὴν ἡλικίαν ἐτύγχανεν ὢν ἔν τε ταῖς ὁσημέ-
ραι πράξεσι πολλὰ ταλαιπωρούμενος· εἰκότως οὖν αὐτῷ τὸ μέλι ταχέως ἐξεχολοῦτο
καὶ ταύτῃ βλαβερώτερον ἦν.

—Galen, *De alimentorum facultatibus* I.1
(VI.470–71K)

καλεῖται δέ τι καὶ σάκχαρον, εἶδος ὂν μέλιτος
πεπηγότος ἐν Ἰνδίᾳ καὶ τῇ εὐδαίμονι Ἀρα-
βίᾳ, εὑρισκόμενον ἐπὶ τῶν καλάμων, ὅμοιον
τῇ συστάσει ἁλσὶ καὶ θραυόμενον ὑπὸ τοῖς

people alter the natural constitution of their bodies through their habits and dietary regimens!). Anyway, of these two people arguing with each other about honey, one was an old man, with a constitution naturally inclined toward the phlegmy and a lazy attitude toward his livelihood and everything else that he engaged in, not least his pre-bath exercises; for this reason, honey was useful for him. The other man was naturally bilious, happened to be in his thirties, and was an extremely hard-working person in all his day-to-day tasks; so, reasonably, honey quickly turned to bile in him and was accordingly rather harmful.

—Galen, *On the Properties of Foodstuffs*

There is also something called sugar, being like a solid honey found on reeds in India and Arabia Felix,[2] similar in structure to salt and crushed between the teeth in the same

ὀδοῦσι καθάπερ οἱ ἅλες. ἔστι δὲ εὐκοίλιον, εὐστόμαχον, διεθὲν ὕδατι καὶ ποθέν, ὠφελοῦν κύστιν κεκακωμένην καὶ νεφρούς.

—Dioscorides, *De materia medica* II.82

Cooked Sweets

ὥσπερ γὰρ αὖ τῷ Σωκράτει γυμνάσιον ἦν οὐκ ἀηδὲς ἡ ὄρχησις, οὕτως ᾧτινι τὸ πέμμα καὶ τὸ τράγημα δεῖπνόν ἐστι καὶ σιτίον, ἧττον βλάπτεται· τὸ δ' ἀπέχοντα τῇ φύσει τὸ μέτριον καὶ πεπληρωμένον ἐπιδράττεσθαι τῶν τοιούτων φυλακτέον ἐν τοῖς μάλιστα.

—Plutarch, *De tuenda sanitate praecepta* 124e–f

Dulcia domestica:
　　Palmulas vel dactilos excepto semine, nuce vel nucleis vel piper tritum infercies.

way as salt. It is good for digestion, good for
the stomach; dissolved in water and drunk,
it benefits an ailing bladder and the kidneys.

—Dioscorides, *Medical Substances*

Cooked Sweets

Just as, for Socrates, dancing was a not
disagreeable form of exercise, in the same
way cake and sweets can count as food
and a meal—and thereby be less harmful!
It is when you have eaten a sufficient and
appropriate meal and are already full that
you should exercise the greatest caution
against indulging in such treats.

—Plutarch, *On Keeping Well*

Recipe for a homemade sweet:

Stuff palm dates or finger dates (pits removed) with nuts, pine nuts, or ground

Sales foris contingis, frigis in melle cocto, et inferes.

Aliter dulcia:

Musteos Afros optimos rades et in lacte infundis. Cum biberint, in furnum mittis, ne arescant, modice. Eximes eos calidos, melle perfundis, compungis ut bibant. Piper aspargis et inferes.

Aliter dulcia:

Accipies similam, coques in aquam calidam ita ut durissimam pultem facias, deinde in patellam expandis. Cum refrixerit, concidis quasi dulcia et frigis in oleo optimo. Levas, perfundis mel, piper aspargis et inferes. Melius feceris, si lac pro aqua miseris.

—*Apicius* VII.11.1, 2, 6

pepper. Sprinkle the outside with salt, fry in cooked honey, and serve.

Another sweet:

Peel the best African sweet apples and soak them in milk. When they have drunk it up, put them in the oven at a low temperature, so they don't dry out. Take them out when they are hot, pour honey over them and prick them so they drink it up. Sprinkle with pepper and serve.

Another sweet:

Take a fine wheat flour, cook it in hot water so that you make the densest porridge possible, then spread it out in a pan. Once it has cooled, cut it up like sweets and fry it in the best oil. Take it out, pour on honey, sprinkle with pepper, and serve. They are even better if you substitute milk for the water.

—*Apicius' Cookbook*

APPENDIX I: FURTHER READING

There is a huge amount of scholarship related to the topics of food and diet in classical antiquity. I select here some titles that will be comparatively accessible to a general audience, both in terms of their technicality and in terms of their price and availability, where possible (a few of the translations are unavoidably more obscure).

For readers seeking more background on food, diet, and medicine in ancient Greece and Rome

Dalby, A. *Food in the Ancient World from A to Z.* London: Routledge, 2003.

Dalby, A. *Siren Feasts: A History of Food and Gastronomy in Greece.* New York: Routledge, 1996.

Erdkamp, P., and C. Holleran, eds. *The Routledge Handbook of Diet and Nutrition in the Roman World.* London: Routledge, Taylor and Francis Group, 2019.

Garnsey, P. *Food and Society in Classical Antiquity.* Cambridge: Cambridge University Press, 1999.

Mattern, S. *The Prince of Medicine: Galen in the Roman Empire*. Oxford: Oxford University Press, 2013.

Nutton, V. *Ancient Medicine*. 3rd ed. London: Routledge, 2024.

Wilkins, J. M., and S. Hill. *Food in the Ancient World*. Malden, MA: Blackwell Publishing, 2006.

For readers wanting to cook like an ancient Greek or Roman

Dalby, A., and S. Grainger. *The Classical Cookbook*. Rev. ed. Los Angeles: J. Paul Getty Museum, 2012.

Faas, P. *Around the Roman Table: Food and Feasting in Ancient Rome*. Translated by S. Whiteside. Chicago: The University of Chicago Press, 2003.

Grainger, S. *Cooking Apicius: Roman Recipes for Today*. Totnes: Prospect Books, 2006.

For readers wishing to read translations of the works excerpted here in their entirety

Apicius' Cookbook

Grocock, C., and S. Grainger. *Apicius. A Critical Edition with an Introduction and an English*

Translation of the Latin Recipe Text Apicius. Totnes: Prospect Books, 2006.

Cato, *On Farming*

Dalby, A. *Cato. On Farming. De Agricultura. A Modern Translation with Commentary*. Totnes: Prospect Books, 2010.

Celsus, *On Medicine*

Spencer, W. G. *Celsus. On Medicine*. 3 vols. Loeb Classical Library. Cambridge, MA: Harvard University Press, 1935–38.

Diocles, *Regimen for Health*

van der Eijk, P. J. *Diocles of Carystus. A Collection of the Fragments with Translation and Commentary*. Leiden: Brill, 2000–2001.

Dioscorides, *Medical Substances*

Beck, L. Y. *Dioscorides. De Materia Medica*. Hildesheim: Olms-Weidmann, 2017.

Galen, *On Mixtures*

Singer, P. N., and P. J. van der Eijk, with the assistance of P. Tassinari. *Galen. Works on Human*

Nature. Volume 1. Mixtures (De Temperamentis). Translated with Introduction and Notes. Cambridge: Cambridge University Press, 2018.

Galen, On the Natural Faculties

Brock, A. J. *Galen. On the Natural Faculties, with an English Translation.* Loeb Classical Library. Cambridge, MA: Harvard University Press, 1916.

Galen, On the Properties of Foodstuffs

Powell, O. *Galen. On the Properties of Foodstuffs. Introduction, Translation, and Commentary.* Cambridge: Cambridge University Press, 2003.

Hippocratic *Regimen*

Jones, W. H. S. *Hippocrates. Volume IV.* Loeb Classical Library. Cambridge, MA: Harvard University Press, 1931.

Hippocratic *Regimen in Health*

Lloyd, G. E. R., J. Chadwick, W. N. Mann, E. T. Withington, and I. M. Lonie. *Hippocratic Writings.* Penguin Classics. London: Penguin Random House, 1984.

FURTHER READING

Pliny the Elder, *Natural History*

Rackham, H., W. H. S. Jones, and D. E. Eichholz. *Pliny the Elder. Natural History*. 10 vols. Loeb Classical Library. Cambridge, MA: Harvard University Press, 1938–63.

Plutarch, *On Keeping Well*

Babbitt, F. C. *Plutarch. Moralia. Volume II*. Loeb Classical Library. Cambridge, MA: Harvard University Press, 1928.

Seneca, *Letters*

Fantham, E. *Seneca. Selected Letters. A New Translation*. Oxford World's Classics. Oxford: Oxford University Press, 2010.

APPENDIX II: GREEK AND LATIN TEXT EDITIONS

The Greek and Latin texts reproduced in this volume, including the cited chapter numbers, follow the scholarly editions listed here. Passages from Galen also cite the standard volume and page numbers from the Kühn edition (K) (C. G. Kühn, ed., *Claudii Galeni Opera Omnia*. 20 vols. Leipzig: C. Cnobloch, 1821–33; reissued, Cambridge: Cambridge University Press, 2011). Some of the texts use common editorial annotations, which can be interpreted as follows:

> <*the letters between these brackets have been added by the editor*>
> [*the letters between these brackets should be ignored*]
> †*there is an unsolved problem with the letters between these symbols*†

APPENDIX II

Apicius' Cookbook

Grocock, C., and S. Grainger. *Apicius. A Critical Edition with an Introduction and an English Translation of the Latin Recipe Text Apicius.* Totnes: Prospect Books, 2006.

Cato, *On Farming*

Dalby, A. *Cato. On Farming. De Agricultura. A Modern Translation with Commentary.* Totnes: Prospect Books, 2010.

Celsus, *On Medicine*

Marx, F. *A. Cornelii Celsi Quae Supersunt.* Corpus Medicorum Latinorum I. Leipzig: Teubner, 1915.

Diocles, *Regimen for Health*

van der Eijk, P. J. *Diocles of Carystus. A Collection of the Fragments with Translation and Commentary.* Leiden: Brill, 2001.

Dioscorides, *Medical Substances*

Wellmann, M. *Pedanii Dioscuridis Anazarbei De Materia Medica Libri Quinque.* Vol. 1. Berlin: Weidmann, 1907.

GREEK AND LATIN TEXT EDITIONS

Galen, *On Good and Bad Juices*

Ieraci Bio, A. M. *Galeno. De Bonis Malisque Sucis.* Naples: D'Auria, 1987.

Galen, *On Mixtures*

Helmreich, G. *Galeni De Temperamentis Libri III.* Leipzig: Teubner, 1904.

Galen, *On the Natural Faculties*

Helmreich, G. *Claudii Galeni Pergameni Scripta Minora.* Vol. 3. Amsterdam: Hakkert, 1967. Reprint, Leipzig: Teubner, 1893.

Galen, *On the Properties of Foodstuffs*

Wilkins, J. *Galien. Tome V. Sur les facultés des aliments.* Paris: Les Belles Lettres, 2013.

Hippocratic *Regimen*

Joly, R., and S. Byl. *Hippocratis De Diaeta.* Corpus Medicorum Graecorum I 2,4. 2nd ed. Berlin: Akademie Verlag, 2003.

Hippocratic *Regimen in Health*

Jouanna, J. *Hippocrate. La Nature de l'homme.* Corpus Medicorum Graecorum I 1,3. 2nd ed. Berlin: Akademie Verlag, 2002.

APPENDIX II

Pliny the Elder, *Natural History*

Rackham, H., W. H. S. Jones, and D. E. Eichholz. *Pliny the Elder. Natural History*. 10 vols. Loeb Classical Library. Cambridge, MA: Harvard University Press, 1938–63.

Plutarch, *On Keeping Well*

Babbitt, F. C. *Plutarch's Moralia. Volume II*. Loeb Classical Library. Cambridge, MA: Harvard University Press, 1928.

Seneca, *Letters*

Reynolds, L. D. *L. Annaei Senecae ad Lucilium Epistulae Morales*. Oxford: Clarendon, 1965.

NOTES

Introduction

1. Plutarch, *On Keeping Well* 137a (τὸ γὰρ παρ' ἰα-
τροῦ πυνθάνεσθαι τί δύσπεπτον ἢ εὔπεπτον αὐτῷ
καὶ τί δυσκοίλιον ἢ εὐκοίλιον οὐχ ἧττον αἰσχρόν
ἐστιν ἢ τὸ πυνθάνεσθαι τί γλυκὺ καὶ τί πικρὸν καὶ
αὐστηρόν).

2. The categories of food presented in Part II of
this book are based on dietary, rather than culinary, groupings, but they are also very loosely
arranged around the order of the courses in a
fancy Roman dinner. One notable exception is
that the appetizer course contained a wider array
of foods than the "relishes" that populate my appetizer section (which were certainly used to
whet the appetite but are also good examples of
the types of things that one might add to bread
to make a simple meal). A more elaborate dinner could have also included meat, seafood, and,

most traditionally, egg dishes in the appetizer course (hence the now proverbial phrase *ab ovo usque ad mala* or "from egg to apples," the Latin equivalent of our "soup to nuts"). For surviving sample menus from Roman entertaining, see Chapter 2 of Faas's *Around the Roman Table* from the further reading list in Appendix I.

3. Mary Beard's *SPQR* (Liveright, 2015) offers an overview of the life and diet of the urban poor in Chapter 11. My guide to the sewers of Herculaneum is Erica Rowan's "Sewers, Archaeobotany, and Diet at Pompeii and Herculaneum," in *The Economy of Pompeii*, ed. M. Flohr and A. Wilson (Oxford University Press, 2016), 111–34.

4. Specifically, Oribasius' *Medical Collections*, a fourth-century CE compendium of the medical wisdom of earlier Greek doctors collected by the personal physician to the Emperor Julian.

Seasonal Eating with Hippocrates

1. The idea that wine is the medically recommended beverage for infants probably seems outrageous to the modern reader, but ancient thinkers may have had their empirical reasons. As we see at

the end of the Diocles passage, ancient Greeks and Romans were aware that the wrong water can make you sick. It was likely in some measure in reaction to this knowledge that the default drink for all ages was ideally wine, diluted to the desired level of potency. However, the reader should not imagine hordes of drunken toddlers; as the author here indicates, the wine these children were drinking was mostly water (whose potential contaminants, the modern eye will recognize, would have been mitigated by the alcohol's antibacterial properties).

Lifestyle Management with Diocles

1. Pennyroyal (*Mentha pulegium*), a toxic member of the mint family, was deployed by ancient doctors for a variety of uses, most notably as a contraceptive; in its guise here as a toothpaste, it would have given the mouth a familiar minty freshness.

2. There was a specialized tool used for scraping dirty oil off of the body called a strigil. Many examples survive archaeologically, and still more were depicted on pottery and in statuary. They are reminiscent of shoehorns in shape (see Fig. 2).

3. Galen helpfully defines these snacks, which could be sweet or savory, as "things eaten after dinner for pleasure while you drink" (τὰ παρὰ τὸ δεῖπνον ἐσθιόμενα τῆς ἐπὶ τῷ πίνειν ἡδονῆς ἕνεκα) (*Alim. Fac.* I.34 [VI.550K]), including everything from fruit, nuts, and sweetened treats to boiled chickpeas and roasted beans (*Alim. Fac.* I.7, 19 [VI.498, 531K]).

4. Aristotle, a rough contemporary of Diocles, tells us (*History of Animals* 5.19 [551a16]) that the Greek words I have translated as "kale" (ῥάφανος) and "cabbage" (κράμβη) are synonyms. Clearly, Diocles intends for his audience to differentiate between them in some way, so I have somewhat arbitrarily assigned each to a different member of the Brassica family. A similar degree of latitude necessarily underlies my translation of most plant names, as discussed in the "Note on the Translations" in the Introduction.

5. A particularly popular member of the dock family, *Rumex patientia* (also called garden patience or monk's rhubarb) is a tangy green similar to spinach.

6. Also known as garden cress, *Lepidium sativum* is a peppery green similar to watercress and mustard greens.

Vegetables and Legumes

1. A small unit of measure, equivalent to about 3 tablespoons.
2. Early in his career, Galen held a salaried position as doctor to a troop of gladiators in his home city of Pergamon (in modern Turkey). Curious readers may consult the list of further reading in Appendix I for Susan Mattern's splendidly readable biography of Galen, which covers his gladiator period in Chapter 3.

Compound Dishes

1. A foraged plant of the fennel family (but speculated to have had more of a funky garlic flavor), silphium was imported from Cyrene in modern Libya and used widely as a seasoning. It was so beloved by the Romans that they ate it into extinction.

NOTES

Fruits, Nuts, and Sweets

1. It was a common belief in antiquity that head lice were the result of spontaneous generation from an excess of moist residues in the head; see, e.g., Aristotle, *Problems* 1.16 (861a10–19), 20.12 (924a6–16).
2. The Roman name (meaning "Blessed Arabia") for the province that encompassed what is now Yemen.